RAJA YOGA

A simplified and practical course

Of all the forms of yoga which are taught and practiced in the East, Raja Yoga is considered the kingly science; it aims at the development of man's full potential and the expression of his inner spiritual self.

In this small volume the author offers the basic technique of this ancient classic system of yoga in a graded practical "do it yourself" course divided into ten lessons. The instructions include posture, breathing, right attitudes and, most importantly, methods of meditation. This simplified course will be of inestimable value in aiding the student to find a means of inner quiet amidst the rush and turmoil of a busy life, to discover new insights and to realize himself as an integrated human being.

Wallace Slater is a British scientist who has spent more than forty years in the study and practice of yoga as part of his daily routine of life. This book on Raja Yoga is a companion volume to his earlier small work *A Simplified Course of Hatha Yoga,* also published as a Quest Book.

RAJA YOGA

A Simplified and Practical Course

by
WALLACE SLATER

A QUEST BOOK

Published under a grant from the Kern Foundation

THE THEOSOPHICAL PUBLISHING HOUSE
Wheaton, Ill., U.S.A.
Madras India/London England

First Published 1968
© V. W. Slater, 1968

Quest Book Edition 1968, published by the
Theosophical Publishing House, Wheaton, Ill.
A department of the Theosophical Society in America,
by arrangement with Theosophical Publishing House,
London Ltd.
Third Quest Book printing, 1975

ISBN: 0-8356-0131-5
Library of Congress Catalog Number 71-3051

Printed in the United States of America

SUMMARY OF THE LESSONS

PREFACE

This simplified Course of Raja Yoga is based on the author's experience in its practice under personal tuition and with the benefit of a wide study of yoga literature. The books on the subject go into great detail on the philosophy of yoga. Many are just commentaries on the *Yoga Sutras of Patanjali*, but they do not give detailed instructions in lesson form. There was therefore a need for a graded practical course for the guidance of those unable to have personal tuition. The book can be one's teacher, the instructions being given in the form of "do this" rather than as vague suggestions.

The Course has been planned to take ten months, one lesson a month. At this rate and going lesson by lesson the reader will absorb the spirit and practice of Raja Yoga with its great benefits almost imperceptibly. Account has been taken of the person who has a minimum of time to devote to the subject but who, nevertheless, wants to take advantage of its benefits and to know how it may be fitted into a daily routine.

Attention is called to the companion book *A Simplified Course of Hatha Yoga*. That form of yoga is concerned with the control of the physical body. Raja Yoga is directed towards the control of the mind. Both practices are of value and one may begin with either according to natural inclination. It is said that all forms of yoga begin with Hatha and end with Raja.

V. W. SLATER

INTRODUCTION

The term yoga is now generally applied to many forms of asceticism, meditation and spiritual training whether practised by Hindus, Buddhists or Christians. It is, however, primarily an ancient Indian form of discipline which has been modified by later Indian writers, adopted by Buddhists and practised in the West in many different forms by people professing the Christian faith or none. It is therefore to India that we look for the original source material.

Yoga, derived from *yuj*, implies "to bind together", "to yoke", and in this sense its practice is to unite the individual spirit of man with the greater Spirit of God (*Ishwara*), or with the Oversoul of humanity. But first there must be an unbinding, a separation of the external from the internal, of the "profane world" from the spirit. This is achieved by various yoga practices which aim to withdraw consciousness from the periphery to the centre, from the material world of our outward senses to a calm inner centre of reality, variously called spirit, truth, wisdom, the Self, *ātma*. At this level man knows that he is one with all humanity and with the Eternal. Yoga may also be regarded as a process for attaining perfection, the goal of normal evolution. According to Radhakrishnan, "the yoga discipline is nothing more than the purification of the body, mind and soul, and preparing them for the beatific vision" (*Indian Philosophy*).

The withdrawal of consciousness from the outer world of the senses may be achieved by control of the physical body in order to open it to the cosmic energy by breathing and physical exercises (Hatha Yoga); by concentrating on the psychic centres to awaken the primordial cosmic energy of the individual (Laya or Kundalini Yoga); by making use of the repetition of certain words and phrases to steady the mind (Mantra Yoga). It may also be achieved by working from the centre to the periphery to effect union of higher and lower by control of thought (Jnana Yoga); by control of one's emotional consciousness through devotion to an ideal (Bhakti Yoga); by control of one's actions from non-selfish motives (Karma Yoga).

These various forms of yoga and others are to be found in the Sanskrit scriptures: the Upanishads, particularly the *Yogatattva*, the *Dhyānabindu* and the *Nādabindu*; the *Mahābhārata*, particularly the added portions, the *Bhagavad Gita* and the *Mokshadharma*; and the *Yoga Sutras* of Patanjali.

The *Yogatattva* recognizes four kinds of yoga: Mantra, Laya, Hatha and Raja; the *Mahābhārata* bases its yoga on direct perception of the mystical aspect of nature, with stress on purity, control of desire and compassion. The *Bhagavad Gita* undoubtedly represents a high point in Indian spirituality, validating all "paths" of union with the highest.

The classic yoga of India is that of Patanjali, which has been recognized by Brahmins as one of the six orthodox systems of philosophy (*darshanas*). This yoga is Raja Yoga and is said to embrace all six yogas mentioned above. It has also been called the Yoga of Will. It has been defined as the earliest and most scientific treatment of the subject of self-transformation, for the attainment of union with the Real, the Eternal. It develops will through concentration and meditation by tuning the nervous system to be in harmony with higher vibrations.

2

The *Yoga Sutras* or *Aphorisms of Patanjali* set out the system of Raja Yoga as eight steps, stages or sub-divisions (*āshtānga*, literally with eight limbs). These are tabulated in his chapter II, sutra 29, as follows, the Sanskrit term being given here with a simple translation for each:

(1)	*Yama*	self-restraint
(2)	*Niyama*	self-discipline
(3)	*Āsana*	posture
(4)	*Prānāyāma*	control of breath
(5)	*Pratyāhāra*	control of the senses
(6)	*Dhāranā*	concentration
(7)	*Dhyāna*	meditation
(8)	*Samādhi*	contemplation

The above translations are expanded in more detail in the lessons that follow.

Textbooks usually treat the subject sequentially in the above order on the principle that each stage depends upon some mastery of the earlier stages. In this Course each lesson embraces several sub-divisions to enable the student to proceed at a steady all-round pace along the several lines of development.

The first two stages are essential preliminary preparation or requirements and deal with morality and ethics. The next three are concerned with the discipline of the body and the senses. The five are thus external preparation (*bahiranga*).

The last three stages are internal (*antaranga*) and cover all aspects of mind control.

The instructions and exercises in this Course are grouped under five headings:

Behaviour. This covers self-restraint and self-discipline, *yama* and *niyama*, and is particularly concerned with the moral and ethical requirements before full yoga practices can be effective or even safe.

Body discipline. This deals with those postures, *āsanas*, used for meditation, but includes general advice for the health of the body by attention to personal hygiene, diet and relaxation.

Breathing. Control of breath, *prānāyāma*.

Sense restraint. Control of the senses, *pratyāhāra*, literally "drawing back", hence restraining the mind from following the impressions of the senses, or freedom from the senses.

Meditation. This is the most important practice in Raja Yoga and covers all aspects of mind control from concentration of thought (*dhāranā*, or exclusive attention to one idea), through meditation (*dhyāna*, or continued attention taken beyond the plane of sensuous perception) to contemplation (*samādhi*, the final fulfilment or state of ecstasy). This threefold process is called *sanyama*, which has been translated as "poise"; its literal meaning is "holding together".

The above classification is used throughout the lessons. The Course is meant to be a practical one to be taken slowly, making sure of the careful practice of each lesson before proceeding to the next one.

Sanskrit terms

Throughout this Course Sanskrit terms have been included because they will help for reference purposes when consulting other books on yoga, some of which use only Sanskrit terms. There is, otherwise, no need to be concerned about them, except in so far as they give a meaning beyond the simple English translation. This will become evident as the Course proceeds.

4

LESSON 1

Behaviour

Yoga is a form of training that must be self-chosen and self-imposed. If the recommendations are followed conscientiously the result can be surprisingly efficient: a healthy body, a one-pointed mind, an awakened intuition.

The aspirant must be prepared to alter his way of life and to give a little time each day to yoga practice. It is useless to embark on such practice if one thinks that life can go on just the same as before. It is therefore important to begin with a consideration of one's natural behaviour, particularly from a moral and ethical point of view. This is because the practice of yoga can stimulate all the activities of our living, and this applies equally to bad habits as to good ones.

So our first lesson begins with the two aspects of behaviour, SELF-RESTRAINT (*yama*) and SELF-DISCIPLINE (*niyama*). On their own they do not constitute yoga, but they are essential preliminary preparation for the practice.

The Sanskrit word *yama* literally means restraint, therefore restraint with regard to one's behaviour, self-restraint. It has been expressed in many ways by different authors: abstention, harmlessness, control or self-control, forbearance, refusal, purification, avoidance. By tradition there are five restraints, which are usually expressed as negations, "thou shalt not":

absention from   i. violence (ৰাংসা)
                    ii. falsehood (সত্য)

iii. stealing (অস্তেয়)
iv. intemperance, sensuality (ব্রহ্মচর্য)
v. acquisitiveness. (অপরিগ্রহ)

These may be expressed positively as:

    i. helpfulness, gentleness
   ii. truthfulness
  iii. uprightness, honesty
   iv. temperance
    v. openhandedness, generosity.

Niyama literally means unrestrained but is interpreted rather as "what one should do", that is, positive action as distinct from the negative restraints of *yama*. Thus it implies how one should behave. The most usual expression in yoga literature is observance, but other interpretations are: ceremony, ritual, obligation, regular habits, non-refusal. We have preferred the term self-discipline. There are five disciplines to be observed or obeyed:

    i. cleanliness (শৌচ)
   ii. contentment (সন্তোষ)
  iii. austerity (তপ)
   iv. self-study (or study of the "ancient wisdom") (স্বাধ্যায়)
    v. devotion to an ideal. (ঈশ্বর প্রণিধান)

In this Course it is proposed to take only one self-restraint and one self-discipline in each of the first five lessons. It is better to take time to improve one's moral and ethical behaviour, rather than to try to force an overall improvement in a time too short for the result to become a natural habit of living. This method is always used by teachers of yoga and ensures a steady progress

6

towards a result that can be maintained throughout life.

Also this Course is meant to be a practical one and simplified. It will therefore give a simple practical approach to each of the behaviour injunctions, without too much theoretical discussion.

Non-violence (ahimsā)

This is the first of the self-restraints. Its elementary form is the injunction "thou shalt not kill", but it goes beyond the usual interpretation of that commandment and includes the non-killing of animal life. It also includes non-injury.

The aspirant should begin by examining his behaviour in terms of a desire not to cause pain to any creature. Desire will then be changed to determination as the wish is expressed in action.

So, for the period of this lesson, begin each day by asking yourself whether your behaviour by thought, word or deed is likely to hurt anyone or to cause them pain, whether that pain be physical, emotional or mental. At the end of the day ask yourself, "Have I done anything to hurt anyone?", and follow this up by the more positive thought, "Have I been kind and helpful to others?"

Begin by thinking of those near to oneself: the family, business associates, tradespeople; then include people you meet but do not know, people you pass in the street, shop assistants; finally, think of those whom you do not even meet but whose letters you may have to answer, or about whom you read in the newspapers.

Proceed slowly, day by day, until an attitude of kindness becomes such a habit that you no longer need to

7

think about it. You will not gossip unkindly about other people; you will not misjudge others' motives.

These suggestions may seem so obvious as to be hardly worth time and effort, but yoga demands meticulous attention to detail.

The above morning and evening exercise refers only to our fellow men. At a later stage we shall extend this to animals: general kindness in the first place and doing them no hurt.

Cleanliness (shaucha)

This is the first of the self-disciplines. Some translations of *Patanjali's Aphorisms* limit this to physical cleanliness, namely personal hygiene. That is only the beginning, the external, and must be accompanied by purification at all levels and particularly purification of the mind by the practice of many virtues. In fact many teachers consider this mental aspect to be of more importance than bodily cleanliness.

Bodily cleanliness means personal external washing, but also includes elimination of residues and impurities from the internal organs: the digestive tract, the lungs, the nasal passages, etc., as given later in this lesson under Body Discipline.

It is therefore proposed that the exercises for this discipline be on the mental aspect, external cleanliness of the whole body being taken for granted as normal for civilized man.

Begin the day as you wash by saying, "Pure thoughts, pure emotions." Thus you will associate the cleansing of the body with the cleansing of the mind and the emotions. Follow this up by a determination that your words during the day shall be pure. All this should result in behaviour that radiates universal love and

8

equanimity. The idea may be helped by pondering on the consequences of mental purity: pleasantness of mind, freedom from thoughts that corrupt or debase, innocence, pleasantness.

Body Discipline

This section includes posture (*āsana*), the third step in raja yoga. The reason given for body discipline immediately after moral and ethical discipline (behaviour) is that it is necessary to eliminate any disturbances of the mind caused by the physical body. Therefore certain postures are recommended, as making the body insensitive to environment and therefore less likely to hinder concentration.

In this Course a wider preparation of the body is included in the hope of making the whole body healthy and more easily controlled. The specific postures or seats for raja yoga will not be dealt with until lesson 3. Hygiene, diet and relaxation will prepare the way. (Hints on diet are given in lesson 2.)

Personal hygiene

Hygiene is a science dealing with the preservation of good health. This means that the practice of personal hygiene should help to avoid illness. Doctors recognize that this should be their first responsibility, the curing of disease being secondary when prevention has failed. A knowledge of the principles of healthy living is an essential preliminary to the practice of yoga.

Such knowledge as is available is imperfect and there are many contradictory schools of thought. Some will insist on a daily cold bath on rising; others recommend hot steam baths followed by heavy massage. There are cults in favour of periods of complete nudity, exposure

9

of the whole body to sun and air. Exercises recommended range from slow graceful rhythmic movement to strenuous physical muscle development.

The suggestions given here are taken from the ancient yoga tradition and are based on the general experience of those interested in healthy living. It must, however, be emphasized that there are no universal rules of hygiene; each individual must find those which suit him, and this will depend on his own idiosyncrasies: age, early training, weight, heredity, constitutional weaknesses, environment and occupation, and so on. Each individual should study how best he can maintain his health; a doctor can help, but ultimately it is a personal responsibility.

The most important principle of hygiene is *cleanliness*, but, from the point of view of yoga, this should be broadened into the efficient elimination of the body's used products. For example, dirt is not necessarily harmful, but regular washing of the whole body is necessary, not just to remove dirt, but to keep the pores of the skin open and to remove bodily impurities eliminated through the pores. For this reason a daily bath is recommended: if at night preferably a warm or hot one, say 90°–98° F or over, as this is relaxing; if in the morning, then a tepid bath 65°–90° F as a mild stimulant. Alternatively a friction bath, using a wet towel over the whole body, will help the skin to eliminate poisons.

Bad teeth can cause harm to the whole body. Soft sugary foods that need no chewing can contribute to dental decay. It is therefore better to brush the teeth after meals or in addition to the early-morning use of the toothbrush.

The nasal passages can be cleansed by sniffing warm

water into the nostrils and expelling it through the mouth. This must be done gently and there must be no violent blowing of the nose as this could cause infection of the tube leading to the ear. Throat trouble is best helped by gargling with a weak solution of common salt, one level teaspoonful in one pint of warm water. This solution can also be used for the nose if water alone causes discomfort.

Internal cleanliness is even more important than external. Regular bowel action should be encouraged by establishing a routine habit at a set time, rather than by the use of aperients. For constipation it is better to use foods containing "roughage", or bran, prunes, figs or dates.

The lungs may be "cleansed" by breathing exercises. The oxygen in the air does the cleansing and therefore deep breathing should be encouraged so as to fill the lungs. This can be done most simply by arranging regular daily walks. If you go to work by car or public transport, walk some of the way.

The above are only suggestions for the individual to work out his own routine. The important point about hygiene in relation to yoga is that it should become a *habit*, a routine of living. A well-ordered blend of habits intelligently formed can lead to a life in which we can exert our full powers unhindered.

Relaxation

The body must have regular periods of relaxation. When travelling in a car or any vehicle, do not sit tensely as if you wished to help the car to move forward, just relax into the seat and let the car do the work on its own. For sleeping use warm bedclothes, but of light weight.

Relaxation posture (*shavāsana*)

This is an exercise particularly used in hatha yoga, but it is a useful addition for all forms of yoga.

Lie flat on the back with the feet slightly apart and relax muscle by muscle from the head downwards, terminating the exercise by tensing each muscle group also from head to toe.

Begin the exercise by breathing in and out slowly and deeply a few times. Then let the whole body go limp. Feel each muscle group relax: eyebrows, mouth, neck, shoulders—and so on to the toes.

Then follow the same course but now tensing each muscle group.

Finally have a good overall stretch.

Do this exercise daily on rising.

Breathing

It is important in all the yogas to include some control of breathing. In raja yoga this control does not mean holding one's breath for long periods, nor does it include the elaborate breathing exercises of hatha yoga. It means learning to breathe steadily, fully and in a relaxed way.

The following exercise, which will be referred to as the **Basic Breath,** should be done daily immediately after the relaxation posture.

Lie flat on the back with hands on the diaphragm, i.e. just below the ribs. *Breathe in* through the nose slowly and as deeply as possible. As the lungs fill, press on the diaphragm to force air into the chest. Fill with air the lower, middle and upper parts of the lungs in that order. Then *breathe out* as slowly as you breathed in, through the nose. Gently draw in the abdomen at the end of the breathing out.

Do this six times, finally expelling the air quickly.

To summarize the practical work for this lesson, allocate, say, 5–10 minutes each morning on:

  i. thinking about non-violence and purity of mind and emotions, the first restraint and the first discipline;
  ii. the relaxation posture;
  iii. the basic breath exercise.

Throughout the day apply the principles of personal hygiene.

The Course has been planned on the basis that each lesson will take one month, but each must determine his own rate.

LESSON 2

Behaviour

Non-falsehood (*satya*)

This is the second of the self-restraints, "not to lie"; the literal meaning of *satya* is truth.

At the level of speech it means we shall not say what we know to be false. Nor shall we mislead others by inferring that we know something when we are only guessing or making dogmatic assumptions. It implies that we shall not make rash hasty judgments. This restraint must, however, be given a much broader meaning: to be true in thought and deed, as well as in word.

The aspirant should begin each day by setting himself the ideal of truthfulness in its very broadest sense. Begin with the thought, "I will be true to myself", "to my Higher Self". Think in terms of the highest principles of which you are capable, and determine that your thoughts and actions shall be in accord with those principles; to be true to one's principles is as high as can be expected, but at least aim that high.

Another point to note is that lying does not refer only to language. We can lie by actions, if those actions mislead others, e.g. to let them think we have done something we neither have done nor intend to do.

At the end of the day ask yourself whether you have kept to the principle of truthfulness. There may be a temptation to try to justify a falsehood; no progress will be made in raja yoga if we succumb to such temptation. We must not mislead ourselves any more than others.

An experienced yogi should be able to say that he has done what is best for the promotion of what is good, so far as his knowledge enabled him to judge.

Contentment (*santosha*)

This is the second of the self-disciplines: "From contentment arises superlative happiness" (*Patanjali* II, 42). It is not just passive acceptance of one's circumstances, but rather an active appreciation of the people by whom one is surrounded, an active appraisal of one's circumstances in order to be able to make the most of them, even if they appear frustrating.

Here also begin the day by thinking about this virtue. Determine to make the best of whatever happens during the day, to be content with both people and events. Make a strong mental image of yourself as a happy and contented individual, looking on the bright side of things, helping others to do the same. During the day remind yourself of your determination, remembering that raja yoga is the yoga of the will, and therefore we can strengthen our will by such determination.

Self-restraints and self-disciplines are virtues on which much theory could be written and studied. But this is a practical course, and the aspirant must practise the virtues in his daily living rather than consider them a philosophical study.

Body Discipline

Diet

What we eat and drink and how we do it has a profound effect on both our physical and mental behaviour. It is therefore necessary to give some consideration to our eating habits. The suggestions here and in lesson 4 must be adapted to the individual. Be wise in what you eat, but do not become so absorbed in the subject that you become a bore to other people and a worry to yourself. Food should be nourishing and not too rich nor over-elaborate.

Eat slowly, so that the digestive juices have a chance to work; digestion begins in the mouth. Do not eat immediately before or after exercise; if you walk to your meal, have a short rest before eating. Similarly, remember that food is not properly digested when taken under emotional or mental stress. For this reason music during the meal can be helpful and this applies especially when eating alone.

Do not live to eat, but eat to live. Food should therefore be simple, nourishing and soothing, leaving no sense of heaviness after the meal.

For drinks, fruit juices are best, and definitely no alcohol should be taken. Tea should be freshly prepared and not too strong. Coffee should not be taken in the late evening as it is then too stimulating. Milk, if taken as a drink, should be sipped and treated as a food.

It is better not to drink during a meal, but an hour or so before or after. Each must, however, decide what suits him best; the particular practice to avoid is that of eating and drinking "at the same time", that is, washing the food down with a drink.

Breathing

A basic breathing exercise was given in lesson 1. It is necessary to understand why breath control (*prānāyāma*) plays an important part in all forms of yoga. In some forms it is taken to extremes so that the automatic natural rhythm is brought under the control of the will, which imposes conscious variations, including the ability to hold one's breath for long periods of time.

In raja yoga control of breath is limited to the harmonizing of the rhythm to a slow steady pace which the body's automatic processes can continue without any effort of the will. Its object is to cleanse the blood and feed the nerves, and to assist in the control of the mind, thereby producing serenity and an inner calm.

Prāna

Prāna literally means breath, but it is taken to mean the life principle at all levels of consciousness: acting, feeling and thinking. *Yāma* is restraint, and so *prānā-yāma* means restraint, or control, of breathing and hence control of the life forces at all levels.

According to the occult tradition, as we breathe in, so we take in the cosmic breath of the Universal Spirit. At the physical level the nervous system is steadied and calmed so that the life currents flow harmoniously. At the mental level the mind is freed from external disturbances so that it can become a channel for the Cosmic Life. This leads to control of the mind, control of the thinking principle, by man's highest principle, the will (*ātma*), sometimes just called the Self.

Cosmic or prāna breathing

With the above background, practise the *basic breath* given in the first lesson, but while breathing in think of the whole body as being filled with a vital force, a health-giving force. At the same time try to sense a surrounding field of force which extends beyond the physical body; this has been called an "etheric double", a "psychic atmosphere" or an aura.

17

When breathing out think of the elimination of impurities so that the body with its aura begins to feel a sense of purity.

Then let your consciousness rest at the mental level, free the mind from its restless agitation, still its constant activity and feel calm and serene.

To summarize the practical work for this lesson:

i. Under behaviour think only about non-falsehood and contentment. Do not try to include the two behaviour injunctions given in lesson 1 as it is better to concentrate on the two given in this lesson.

ii. The relaxation posture (lesson 1).

iii. The basic breath, as given in lesson 1, with the additional associated thinking, as given in this lesson.

LESSON 3

Behaviour

Non-stealing (asteya)

This is the third of the self-restraints, not taking other people's property by stealth or force, not to steal. At the mental level this also means non-covetousness.

As with the other injunctions, this must be given a very broad meaning. "Thou shalt not covet." It is first the desire to possess what other people have that leads to the active taking of their possessions. But the mere thought of coveting what other people have upsets one's emotional and mental equilibrium. It makes one feel dissatisfied, envious. The actual theft, if it should result, is a mere by-product of the original thought.

The yogi reduces his physical needs to the possessions he can use, and even those he holds lightly. He does not acquire things for the sake of having them, but only if actually needing them. He finds pleasure in seeing other people enjoy their possessions, and he does this without any sense of jealousy.

Renunciation is another aspect of this injunction. If we do not covet another's possessions, we can equally let go of our own. This includes freeing ourselves from desires: desire for power, for pleasure, for excitement, for occult powers. The *Bhagavad Gita* here includes "renunciation of the fruits of one's acts".

No one beginning to practise yoga is likely to be tempted to steal in the crude sense. So, to be practical, concentrate on the development of a state of mind free from covetousness. Begin the day by thinking that what you possess is held in trust for the work you have to do. You will use your possessions for the service of others. You are happy to know that others can enjoy their possessions.

At the end of the day ask yourself whether you have felt at all dissatisfied to see others apparently "better off" than you are in worldly goods. And then realize that all worldly possessions are but temporary. They do not belong to the spirit.

Austerity (tapas)

This is the third of the self-disciplines. The Sanskrit word *tapas* comes from the verb *tap* meaning "to heat" or "to burn". Thus it means having a burning desire to achieve one's goal and a readiness to undergo self-discipline for this purpose. It has been translated as devotion. Austerity implies asceticism, but it is better to think of it as ardour, that is, ascetic only in the sense of being prepared to undergo self-deprivation in order to achieve a desired result, just as an athlete forgoes certain pleasures in his training.

This discipline particularly leads to the development of will-power, determination to succeed and, in yoga, a regular daily practice, without excuse or complaint, of the whole discipline recommended.

Austerity develops strength of character, moral courage, a well-disciplined body, a mind balanced in joy or sorrow.

Here are two exercises that will help to establish this quality in the would-be yogi:

    i. Decide for a given period to go without some plea-sure, such as sugar in the tea, sweets, biscuits. This will give a sense of satisfaction that one is not a slave to habit.

ii. Decide for a few days to get up at an earlier hour than usual. Set the time and then keep to it. Use an alarm clock if necessary, but when it goes, get out of bed at once without hesitation.

You can think of other exercises; the idea is to decide to do something requiring a definite act of will to overcome one's natural inclination.

Body Discipline

Postures (āsanas)

Āsana means a seat, but in hatha yoga it includes a wide range of physical exercises in the nature of postures for bending and stretching the trunk and limbs. In raja yoga we are concerned only with postures that can be used when meditating, that is, the sitting postures.

During meditation it is important to eliminate any disturbance of the mind that the body may cause. The posture must be such as to render the body insensitive to environment.

The most natural posture for the human form is to sit cross-legged on the floor or on a cushion, and in India and many other countries this is the regular custom. In Western countries children will do this naturally, but as they grow up and use chairs their limbs lose the necessary elasticity.

Three cross-legged postures will be given for those who wish to try them, but it is more important to use a comfortable posture than to try to force one that is uncomfortable. The important point is that the spine shall be erect and free, not lounging in an easy chair. The chest must be in a position for easy breathing. A posture using a chair is introduced for Western students

21

who cannot sit cross-legged: this we have called the Egyptian posture.

Simple cross-legged posture (*sukhāsana*)

This is the "pleasant seat".

Sit on a rug with the legs out in front. Bend the left leg at the knee and place the left foot under the right *thigh*, sole upwards and with the left knee as near the ground as possible. Do not worry if your knee cannot touch the ground.

Now bend the right leg at the knee and place the right foot under the left *leg*, sole tilted up. Note that for this simple posture the right foot is under the left leg, not the left thigh. The knees will probably be 4–6 inches from the ground.

Keep the body erect and extend the arms outwards to rest the back of the wrists on the knees.

Some people prefer to reverse the order, i.e. to have the right foot under the left thigh for the first movement.

The above description is rather detailed. If you find it easy to sit cross-legged on the ground, then ignore these instructions and just take the most comfortable position for yourself, so long as you keep the body erect.

The position of the hands is that for an "open meditation". For a "closed meditation" the hands may rest centrally one on the other with palms up, or with the fingers interlaced.

Egyptian posture

This is not found in the Indian tradition but is introduced in the Course for the benefit of Westerners and for elderly students.

Sit naturally on an upright chair, with or without a cushion. Have the feet and legs slightly apart and the spine upright. It is preferable not to lean on the back of the chair, but to let the hands give whatever support is necessary. The hands may be palms downwards or upwards on the thighs, or one hand resting on the other. Or the hands may be clasped, palms up. The head must be upright, not dropping forward.

The height of the chair is important. It should be such that the feet rest squarely on the floor with the thighs horizontal. If the chair is too high the seat will press on the sciatic nerve and cause discomfort and may stop the blood-flow. If too low it may cause cramp and jerks in the thigh muscles.

Breathing

Regular deep (rhythmic) breathing

Sitting in either the simple cross-legged posture or the Egyptian posture, breathe in and out steadily through the nose, keeping a regular rhythm—that is, the same time for breathing in as for breathing out. The idea is to avoid erratic timing. If you time yourself you will probably find that you breathe in for 2–3 seconds and then out for 2–3 seconds. This gives 12–15 respirations per minute; you may find you do 15 to 18 per minute

Most people's breathing is shallow and erratic. Your first job is to make it regular, and then deep. Deep breathing means a slower rate, so begin by extending the time for in-breathing to 4 seconds, and out for 4 seconds. Then go to 5, then to 6 and finally to 7 seconds, giving a final respiration rate of only 4–5 per minute. However, proceed slowly, do not try to go to the final slow rate in one session, take several days or even weeks. It is more important to establish steady, regular and rhythmic breathing at your natural rate than to make the rate slower. There is no need to use a watch for timing; just count one, two, three—slowly.

The idea of breathing more slowly is for your meditation periods rather than for regular use.

To summarize the daily practical work for this lesson:

i. Under behaviour proceed with non-stealing (non-covetousness) and austerity as you have with the injunctions of behaviour in lessons 1 and 2, that is, resolution in the morning and a look back at the end of the day.

ii. The relaxation posture.

iii. The basic breath as given in lesson 1 and *without* the additional ideas given in lesson 2. Those additional ideas about *prāna*, taking in the vital force during the breathing exercise, should now be used only when doing breathing exercises in one of the postures where the spine is upright.

iv. Try out the simple cross-legged and Egyptian postures to decide which you will adopt, and then practice regular deep breathing as given in this lesson, using the posture you have chosen.

LESSON 4

Behaviour

Non-sensuality (*brahmacharya*)

This is the fourth of the self-restraints, not to be sensual. Or put as an injunction, to exercise self-restraint in all things, but especially with regard to sexual appetite.

Most books on yoga translate the word *brahmacharya* as "chastity in thought, word and deed", celibacy or sexual abstinence. It is derived from *brahma*, the supreme All-Soul, and *charyā* meaning external acts of worship. Thus the combined word literally means worship of the Supreme Being and is therefore more correctly interpreted as a "life of holiness, especially religious studentship" (or probation) (*A Sanskrit Primer*, E. D. Perry, Columbia Univ. Press, 1936). Its broad meaning is therefore a life of sacred study, a devotion for divine wisdom and learning (*Sanskrit Keys to the Wisdom Religion*, Judith Tyberg, Point Loma, 1940). A simple translation is "spiritual conduct" (*Yoga*, Ernest Wood, 1959).

The above explains why advanced books on yoga point out that this self-restraint is a state of mind and has little to do with whether one is married or unmarried. We are told that almost all yogis of ancient India were married men with children, who did not shirk their social responsibilities.

Thus in practising this self-restraint think of it as self-control in all things. Be temperate in eating, in sexual relations, in movement, in emotional expression, in thought. Avoid excesses of all kinds. Be gentle in action and speech. Such behaviour will prepare the aspirant for subsequent practice in advanced meditation, and he will, at the same time, be an influence for peace in his surroundings.

Let these thoughts be with you, as a background throughout the day, using the keywords: temperance, moderation, gentleness.

Self-study (swādhyāya)

This is the fourth of the self-disciplines. *Swa* as a prefix means "one's own"; *dhyāya*, to repeat, to think or to ponder. Hence the complete word means "thinking about one's self", introspection in the sense of getting to know one's own character, one's strength, one's weaknesses.

Spend some time each morning studying your own nature as distinct from the study of the outside world. Who are you? What is your place in the world and what does the world expect of you? What are your failings and how can you correct them? Can you distinguish self from Self, the former associated with selfishness, the latter being selfless?

Body Discipline

Postures (continued)

The following postures for meditation are given for advanced students and for those who find it easy to sit cross-legged. It does not matter if you cannot do them—they are more for reference purposes.

Advanced cross-legged posture (siddhāsana)

This is "the adept's seat".
Begin as for simple cross-legged. Bend the left knee

and, with the help of the right hand, place the left heel under the centre of the pelvis (the perineum). The sole of the left foot will then be touching the inside of the right thigh.

Now bend the right knee, lift the right foot over the left leg and fit the toes snugly into the crevice between the calf and thigh of the left leg.

The position is similar to the simple one but more tightly held, and with the knees definitely resting on the ground. The right foot is higher, its upper surface resting inverted on the left calf.

Hands are now usually held together, palms up, right on left.

Lotus posture (*padmāsana*)

Padma is the lotus, hence the lotus seat. It is the most difficult and not regarded as suitable for Western people. You may, however, wish to know how it is done in case you are young enough to try it. Put briefly, the feet are pulled up so that their top surfaces rest on the thighs.

Begin with the feet out in front. Bend the left knee and bring the heel under the centre of the pelvis as for the advanced posture. Then bring the right foot over the left thigh in an inverted position. Thus the sole of the left foot rests against the underside of the right thigh, while the top of the right foot rests on the top of the left thigh. This is the simple form of the lotus posture.

For the full lotus posture the left foot is pulled between the calf and thigh of the right leg so that the tops of both feet rest on the tops of the thighs.

The hands are then rested on the knees. An official position is to have the hands palms upwards, and with the thumb and forefinger forming a circle, but many people prefer to have the palms downwards on the knees or thighs.

Diet

General hints on diet were given in lesson 2. It should be noted that most yogis follow a vegetarian diet, that is, no meat, fish or poultry. The following hints are given for those who wish to adopt this practice.

As a general rule, natural foods are preferred to processed food, but some people cannot digest salads after the midday meal. Honey, milk, vegetables and fresh fruit make a good basis, but there must be adequate protein, such as eggs, cheese, legumes or nuts taken in moderation.

The following are a few suggestions for newcomers to a vegetarian diet. Adequate nourishment may be obtained by adding an egg, some grated cheese or milled nuts to a plate of vegetables or salad, but this could prove monotonous and uninteresting. There are now many recipe books available giving simple meatless dishes, and a trial of some of these may open the way to a surprisingly interesting diet, without too much trouble.

With regard to protein, one must experiment to find which types suit one's own gastric idiosyncrasies. Try eggs, cheese, nuts, pulses (peas, beans, lentils) or wheat protein (gluten) to find out which are easily digested.

The use of extracts of yeast or of vegetables add piquancy to many dishes. Anyone starting out on a non-flesh diet should aim at having enough interesting food without having to spend too much time on its preparation. Above all, try not to have dull food. Bread and cheese and a tomato may provide sufficient food value, but would not make for a vigorous, healthy life if taken too frequently.

If you cannot manage a strict vegetarian diet, then you may like to try cutting out all red meat, limiting yourself to fish and poultry, or better still to fish only.

Breathing

In lesson 1 a basic breath was given to increase the capacity of the lungs, or rather to ensure that the lungs were used to their full capacity. This was performed lying flat on the back.

In lesson 2 you were told how to associate the cosmic life currents with your breathing, and in lesson 3 you were given instructions how to breathe regularly and deeply for use during meditation. It was suggested that the advice on cosmic or *prāna* breathing should be used with the deep breathing of lesson 3.

This completes what is necessary as far as breathing exercises are concerned for raja yoga. However, some schools of raja yoga, such as that of Shankarāchārya, do recommend another exercise, breathing through alternate nostrils as given below.

Bellows breath (*bhastrika*)

This can be done in the Egyptian posture or in any of the three cross-legged postures. The left hand should rest across the lap, palm up.

Use the right hand to control the nostrils, the thumb on the right nostril and the third finger on the left nostril.

Prepare by *exhaling through the right* nostril, using slight pressure of the finger to close the left nostril. Then *inhale through the right* nostril. Then *exhale through the left* nostril followed by *inhaling through the left*, then *exhaling through the right*.

The timing should be reasonably quick but full. Take twice as long to exhale as to inhale.

The complete cycle should be repeated three times, making six breaths, thus:

> Out right,
> in right, out left,
> in left, out right,
> in right, out left,
> in left, out right,
> in right, out left,
> in left, out right.

The above exercise should be regarded as supplementary and not necessarily part of raja yoga training. It is given as a matter of interest and because some people may like to try it.

Breathing exercises help meditation because they eliminate the disturbances caused by irregular breathing and they soothe the nerves. According to Indian tradition their real purpose is to assist the flow of the vital life force, *prāna* of lesson 2, to bring about the bridging of physical plane consciousness with the life of the higher principles. They thus prepare the mind for meditation practices, which constitute the main body of raja yoga.

The peculiar value of the bellows breath is that it directs *prāna* to the occult centres of the body, but this is of more interest in laya yoga (see Introduction).

Sense Restraint (*pratyāhāra*)

This is the fifth step of the raja yoga tradition (see Introduction, p. 3) and is the final preparation for meditation. The Sanskrit word is derived from *prati*, back, and *āhri*, to bring; thus the whole word is "bringing back", or withdrawal.

It is sometimes translated as abstraction, as when we say "he looked abstracted", meaning that he was withdrawn in thought, or not paying attention, absent-minded. This gives some idea of the full meaning, namely that the mind is withdrawn from the outside world, from the objects of the senses. We are dominated by the exterior world through our senses. Sense restraint is freeing ourselves from that domination.

Steady breathing (*prānāyāma*) prepares for control of the senses because it eliminates erratic behaviour, that is, behaviour that irritates the body and encourages a restless mind, driven hither and thither by the changing impacts of the senses.

The training for this stage of yoga is to learn to control (restrain) the sense organs so that they cease to disturb the mind by their constant stimulation from the outside world. Raja yoga is the yoga of will, and we therefore have to bring our senses under the control of the will before we proceed to the next stage, concentration leading to meditation.

This requirement will be readily understood by any student. No subject can be studied properly, not even the reading of a novel, if one is constantly listening to other people or looking out of the window to see what is happening.

In this lesson we begin by taking the senses of sight, smell and taste.

31

Sight

Look around and realize the wonders of sight. Through the eyes you travel out of the body to the distant horizon. You travel across space to the stars.

Now let your thoughts wander from what you have been looking at, become abstracted, let yourself daydream. Keep your eyes open all the time but stop paying attention to what they see.

You will have experienced this abstraction with yourself and with others when, for example, you have been so preoccupied that you have not noticed what someone else in the room has been doing. Someone may even have removed something from the table in front of you, and you have not noticed.

Then close your eyes and feel the experience of "just being a mind". You are now living in a thought world. Your mind's eye now sees only what is in the mind.

At this point think of a quality such as gentleness or tolerance or sincerity. You are now "looking" with the mind's eye at something that is so within that it is not even the memory of an external sight.

Then open the eyes and look around again.

This exercise will have demonstrated how sense restraint, so far as seeing is concerned, can prepare one to use the mind *at its own level*.

Smell and taste

Begin, as with sight, by experiencing pleasant smells (take a perfume, for example) and enjoyable flavours (taste something you really enjoy). One way of bringing both senses into activity is to smell food being cooked.

32

Then, while the smell and taste are still there, think of something quite different, something in which you are so interested that your attention is distracted from the perfume, or the flavour, or the food. For example, think of a very happy holiday you have had, or of a play you have seen, or of something very pleasant you are going to do tomorrow.

If you are successful you will have forgotten all about the smell or the taste. You are again in the thought world.

As a variation you can think about quite a different smell, say incense, or of a different taste, and allow the memory of that to eliminate the actual smell or taste that your physical sense is experiencing.

There are many ways in which one can exercise the will to restrain these two senses. Just experiment for yourself, realizing that this is only a step towards mental concentration, which we shall begin in the next lesson.

Sanskrit

In the Introduction it was pointed out that Sanskrit terms would be introduced for reference purposes. It will by now be realized that they have had a value. By examining the root origin of the terms and their subtle meanings we have been able to form a clearer idea of the original intention of the various aspects of yoga practice.

The **Exercises** for this lesson should be:

Behaviour. Consideration of non-sensuality (temperance) and self-study (knowing yourself) on lines similar to those recommended for the behaviour injunctions in the earlier lessons.

Body discipline. The relaxation posture.

33

Breathing. (*a*) The basic breath.

        (*b*) Regular rhythmic breathing, increasing the time for each respiration and using the posture chosen.

        (*c*) The bellows breath if you feel like experimenting with this exercise.

Sense restraint. Control of the senses of sight, smell and taste.

LESSON 5

Behaviour

We now come to the last of the self-restraints and self-disciplines, five of each. These make ten injunctions for behaviour. For the period of this lesson concentrate on the two given here. Thereafter you are advised to keep all ten in mind as a code of behaviour. They are not yoga, as such, but they are a necessary preliminary.

The practice of raja yoga strengthens will-power and this can be used for selfish as well as for unselfish ends. It is for this reason that the old teachers insisted on this preliminary ethical and moral discipline. Such discipline itself tests and strengthens the aspirant's will-power and then ensures that the strengthening of that power shall not lead to selfish ends or to the unbalance of the individual's personality. In early times aspirants were not given the later stages until they had satisfied the teacher (*guru*) that they could obey the restraints and observe the disciplines.

After this lesson you may like to establish a routine of thinking about a different injunction each month. Remember, however, that these ten injunctions are but examples for good behaviour. The yogi does not limit his conduct, but recognizes that by the elimination of the crudest forms of evil tendencies he will become aware of subtler forms to be eradicated later.

Non-acquisitiveness (*aparigraha*)

This is the fifth of the self-restraints, non-greed, not to be avaricious. The Sanskrit word is derived from *graha*, grasping or grabbing, and *pari*, all round; the "*a*" makes it negative, "non". It has been translated as not to hoard, or not to collect. It is therefore another aspect of non-stealing or non-covetousness (see p. 19). Non-stealing is not taking what one does not need, non-acquisitiveness is not hoarding what one does not need.

It is elaborated to include not accepting anything without working for it, not to accept favours, not to be attached to possessions, not to accumulate goods.

By this restraint, life becomes simple. There is never any feeling of discontent through lack or loss of anything. Without suggesting that one should expect any reward (in fact such would be quite contrary to yoga practice), it can be said that many people who take up yoga find that everything they *really* need comes to them just when it is needed. They reach a state of mind to be satisfied with whatever happens, because they have a sense of inner security.

For the morning consideration of this restraint, think that it is not what we have but how we use it that is really important. So determine to use what you have for the helping of others, whether those possessions be goods, abilities or qualifications. We are not here to satisfy our own desires.

Devotion to an ideal (*ishwara pranidhāna*)

This is the fifth of the self-disciplines: *Ishwara*, God or the Lord; *pranidhāna*, devotion without ceasing or self-surrender. Yoga is theistic and postulates the existence of a supreme God, *Ishwara*, but this is not a personal god. *Ishwara* means the ruler and is applied to the lord of any hierarchy, including the principles of man. Thus it not only refers to the Supreme Being of the universe but also to the divine Self of man, the Cosmic Spirit in man (*ātma*), his highest principle.

The discipline has therefore been expressed broadly as devotion to an ideal. Theists may prefer the expression "attentiveness to God". Others may prefer surrender to one's highest Self.

The implication of these three ways of expressing it are: an acceptance that the hand of a supreme director is in every event whether that director be an external god or one's inner Self; an acceptance of all experience without resentment; seeing good in everything; an alert attention to one's highest ideal; the disappearance of self in the good of the whole and the dedication of all actions to the divinity within.

In the early-morning practice, as, for example, during the breathing exercises, make an act of dedication. Dedicate yourself to the highest of which you are capable, recognize that there is a purpose behind manifestation and feel prepared to accept whatever the day may bring.

Sense Restraint

Hearing

This sense is not so easy to shut off as sight. We can of course shut it off by plugging the ears, but that is not a natural shutting-off. Sense restraint means that we draw attention away from the organ of sense, while that organ is still exposed to the impacts of the outside world. In lesson 4 we saw how this could be done for sight, even with the eyes open.

For hearing, just sit comfortably and listen to the sounds around you: a clock, birds, the wind, people outside, an acroplane. The more quiet we are, as in the middle of the night, the louder the noises appear; we then begin to hear sounds which we had never noticed before. Let yourself enjoy the wonders of hearing.

Then decide that these sounds are no longer going to activate your thoughts. They are unimportant. Let them flow over you in mass, without trying to pick out the individual noises.

Think in memory about some sound you have enjoyed: music, the sea. Local sounds will then fade into the background.

At this point let the mind listen to that inner voice, the "voice of the silence" which speaks without sound. Feel yourself "in tune with the infinite".

After a short time come back into consciousness; slowly let the ears pick up the local sounds again.

Another useful exercise on sound control is to listen to an orchestra and to pick out particular instruments: the violins, or the piccolos, or the trombones. Or in a room full of people pick out just one person and listen to him.

If the mind can eliminate ten simultaneous sounds and only pay attention to the eleventh, then it should also be able to suppress all eleven simultaneous sounds and pay attention only to one's inner thoughts.

School children are often seen doing their homework in the family surroundings, and they seem able to ignore the conversations around them. See if you can do the same.

Touch

The five senses have been taken in what has been regarded as the order in which they are easy or difficult to restrain. Touch is the most difficult. There is no physical means of suppressing it short of a local anaesthetic.

Sit in a comfortable chair; later repeat the following in the Egyptian or cross-legged posture. You can feel the seat of the chair, the floor. Your hands are resting on something you also feel. The legs, the arms touch the body or each other; at first you hardly notice, but very soon you find you want to move them, to get more comfortable, to relieve the pressure. You feel or imagine you feel an irritation or an itching somewhere, most likely on the face, and you want to put your hand to the spot; or if it is on the neck or body you want to wriggle.

All this realization of the sense of touch will demonstrate that the desire to move, the inability to stay still, is due to what are popularly called "nerves". People looking at you will say you are nervy, or overwrought. In fact it is due to the nervous system being taut; that system includes the sensory nerves and the nerves feeding the muscles.

Therefore continue in the same position but relax your muscles. You have already practised such relaxation in the relaxation posture of lesson 1. A few deep breaths will help. If you resist the desire to move, you may make the tension worse. It is better to admit that you are not comfortable and to move in order to ease yourself into a more comfortable position.

Then sit still for 5 minutes. Teach the body to ignore and then to become unaware of all the little itches and prickles which the physical elementals use to draw attention to themselves. Think of something in which you are keenly interested.

This exercise is a preparation for meditation, so continue, say 5 minutes a day, for several days or even weeks until you really can say that the physical body, particularly its sense of touch, is under control.

Meditation in General

We are now ready to begin meditation, the principal exercise in raja yoga. If you have followed and practised the advice in the first four lessons you will not find meditation too difficult. Otherwise it is better to go back to the beginning again before proceeding farther in this Course. You will then have gained some control under the various headings:

Behaviour, over your general conduct and attitude to life, your character will have been strengthened and you will have a more contented attitude to life in general.

Body Discipline and Breathing, over your body by postures and by the attention you have given to personal hygiene and eating habits. The breathing exercises will have helped to steady the whole nervous system.

Sense Restraint, over your senses. The organs of sense look outwards, in meditation you are going to look within.

The above preparation was designed so that neither body, nor feelings and emotions, nor senses shall disturb the mind when you come to meditate.

There are three stages in what is generally called meditation, the sixth, seventh and eighth steps of formal yoga: concentration, meditation and contemplation (see Introduction, p. 4).

It has been usual for the pupil to be expected to achieve some degree of success in each earlier stage

40

before proceeding to a later stage. In this Course it is recommended that you proceed at the same rate as you have done for the first four lessons, that is, taking two to four weeks for each lesson, preferably four weeks.

This means that you will not be proficient in concentration before proceeding to meditation, and you will be trying contemplation before you have perfected either concentration or meditation. But after you have worked through the three stages for the first time, you should go back to concentration and work through them again at the same rate. Do this again and again; each time you will become more adept.

The reason for this method of working is that, if you spend too long in the first instance on concentration, you may find yourself held up by intellectual concentration as a purely mental exercise, which may not suit your temperament.

By trying all three stages over not too long a period of time, you will discover your own strengths and weaknesses. You may actually find that contemplation comes more easily for you than concentration. There is a danger in this approach and that is that meditation might become no more than an emotional bath, and that is why in the past so much emphasis has been put on the concentration stage. Keep this in mind and avoid letting the contemplation stage become too emotional.

Concentration (*dhāranā*)

This stage is one of giving exclusive attention to one idea. You select an object or an idea and focus your mind on it, you give it your sole attention. The Sanskrit word *dhāranā* is derived from the verb root *dhri* which means to direct one's attention, to maintain, to resolve.

41

Choose a time each day when you can sit down and practice meditation. The word meditation is used for both the whole process covering all three stages and for the second stage (i.e. the seventh step of formal yoga). It should be obvious when reference is made to the second stage only. Suppose you say you will meditate for 5 minutes (a good time to begin with). Then for this 5 minutes you are simply *not interested* in the 101 things that normally occupy your mind. You have all the rest of the day to attend to them. Say to yourself, "This one thing I do, this one thing alone" and then proceed to meditate on the subject selected.

By way of introduction try the following exercise:

Sit cross-legged or Egyptian fashion, close the eyes, breathe naturally and calmly. Feel at peace with the world. Say to yourself, "My body is not the Self. I withdraw my consciousness from my body." Pause and feel the meaning of these statements.

Then say to yourself, "I am not my emotions." Pause and feel the emotions as calm sympathy for others.

Then say, "I am thinking these thoughts, but the Self is higher than the mind. I will control my thoughts." Pause, realize that one's thinking can be controlled and then feel that relaxed sensation when thought itself ceases.

After a short "enjoyment" of this sensation, take a few deep breaths and feel the life of the higher Self flowing into the mind, the emotions, the body—and rise with the sense of being in control of your vehicles of outer consciousness.

This exercise, which has been suitable for general meditation, gives a typical opening and closing for any meditation period, so you can now proceed with a few exercises more particularly on concentration.

Concentration on an external object. Choose your own object from the following list: triangle, square, circle, cube, sphere (ball), an ornament (choose a simple one which you can have before you), a cup, an apple, a flower. You can use a different object each time.

Now seat yourself, Egyptian posture or cross-legged. Make sure the body is comfortable and relaxed, and that you are in a state of sense restraint. With the eyes closed take a few deep breaths. As you will always begin meditation in this way, these instructions will not be given again except as an occasional reminder.

In this exercise you will use the sense of sight, so open your eyes and look at the object you have chosen. Let us assume it is an apple.

Now think of nothing except the apple for 1-3 minutes. This is quite long enough for a beginning. You may be able to go to 5 or 10 minutes later.

Look at the apple. Note its shape, its colour, the stalk. If your mind wanders to the table on which it rests, or to other fruit if it is in a fruit bowl, come back again to the apple. You are interested only in the apple. In looking at the apple, let the eyes blink, do not just stare at it without letting the eyelids drop as that can lead to self-hypnosis. At this stage of concentration you do not want to lose conscious control. You must not drift into a dreamy state. You are looking at the apple and this is your great interest, your sole interest.

Now close your eyes and continue to visualize the apple, to think about it. It is at this point that you may find thoughts wandering: apple, fruit, vegetarianism. Come back to the apple and again you may wander: apple, tree, pruning, roses, garden. Come back to the apple.

Stop before the brain gets tired. Do not strain so that you get a headache or get bored with the exercise.

At the end of the exercise, take a few deep breaths, open the eyes and look around, feel bright and ready for your next job.

Concentration on an internal object. This exercise uses an object that is part of ourselves, such as the tip of the tongue, or the nose, a central point on the top of the head, the area between the eyebrows or the little finger.

Having prepared yourself as usual, begin with the sense of touch. Feel your consciousness withdrawing from the rest of the body to the spot chosen, say the little finger. Wriggle it so that you feel its movement. Hold it still but keep your consciousness there. Think about it, its shape, the three parts with two joints, the fingernail, the sensitivity at the tip.

You can make quite a game of this exercise in concentration, by thinking you are just that finger and nothing else.

Here again, do not keep on too long, and when you decide to stop, do this by allowing consciousness to flow back into the whole hand and so to the rest of the body.

Concentration on an idea. This exercise uses an abstract idea, something without physical form, such as the emotions, the intellect, serenity, a science such as botany, language, or a virtue such as sympathy. The advantage of choosing a virtue is that it can arouse enthusiasm and devotion, and it will build the virtue into one's character.

As this is for the stage of concentration you must not let the mind wander off or around the subject; that will come when you meditate. You might begin with sympathy and at this stage just try to feel the virtue in yourself. It is said that one-pointedness can be achieved more quickly with the feelings than with thought. So take advantage of this and induce an intense concentration of the feeling of sympathy; the mind will then follow the feeling.

Finish this exercise as usual by a few deep breaths and a bright return to the world around.

Special note on concentration. Remember that these exercises are only mental gymnastics, although they can be entertaining and interesting if taken in the right spirit. The mind is exercised in this manner as a step towards meditation and contemplation when the higher states of consciousness may be experienced and when the mind itself will be transcended. This is why advanced meditation is sometimes called transcendental meditation.

Daily Practice

By now you should have decided to allocate 10–15 minutes each day for yoga practices. The early morning is the best time, immediately after rising and after one's regular daily personal hygiene, but you will have to decide when is best for you with regard to your household and business responsibilities. You should not practise yoga immediately after a meal or late at night.

At this stage and for this lesson the following is suggested:

Behaviour. Consider non-acquisitiveness and devotion to an ideal as suggested in this lesson.
Body discipline. The relaxation posture.

Breathing. (*a*) The basic breath.

                  (*b*) Regular rhythmic breathing, increasing the time for each respiration. Do not go beyond 7 seconds in and 7 seconds out (lesson 3).

                  (*c*) The bellows breath (lesson 4) if desired.

Sense restraint. Control of the senses of hearing and touch.

Meditation. Concentration stage: do one of the exercises given in this lesson each day.

LESSON 6

Sense Restraint

In the last two lessons you learnt to withdraw consciousness from the senses, to fix attention in the mind undisturbed by the impact of the outside world.

There is another aspect of this freeing of ourselves from the domination of the senses, namely control of the senses in a positive manner. As well as being able to suppress the senses, we should be able to direct them as indicated below.

The *eyes*, the organs of vision, should be trained to observe accurately so that, when the eyes are closed, we can make a mental picture of what we have observed. This will be done as part of the training in concentration.

The *nose*, the organ of smell, can also be trained to become more sensitive. In suppressing the sense of smell for the purpose of awakening higher consciousness, we should not dull the sense itself. Enjoy pleasant smells, flowers, the smell of the country or of the sea. This can help to take one's consciousness away from the material world into a happy state of bliss. That is why incense is used for religious ceremonies and why some people use it when they are meditating. As one advances in yoga one is able to reproduce the smell of incense at the mental level without actually using it at the physical level. Experiment along these lines, learn how to cut off a smell, how to enjoy a smell and how to create one mentally.

47

The *tongue*, the organ of taste, can be used in a similar way. Enjoy refined flavours; do not spoil your sense of taste by the excessive use of strong flavours such as salt, pepper, sugar. Learn to recognize and appreciate delicate flavours. Having been taught how to suppress the sense of taste, you must also know how to use it correctly. Taste, and this also applies to smell, plays an important part in the assimilation of food by stimulating the digestive juices. A refined sense of taste can lead to the right choice of food, that which is best for the health and well-being of the body.

The *ears*, the organs of hearing, should be trained to be alert. Pay attention to the people around you, listen to them with interest. Listen to the voice of Nature in the garden, or in the country away from the noise of town-life. The advanced yogi in a state of inner alertness will sometimes "hear" sounds from higher levels of consciousness. Listen to that inner voice, it can give inspiration, encouragement and sometimes advice.

The *skin*, the sense of touch, covers a wide area. It should be treated with care. According to the occult tradition, the whole body is surrounded by a field of vital energy which extends about one-quarter of an inch beyond the skin when in a state of "rest", but normally it extends several inches. As a field of force it may be compared with the magnetic field surrounding a magnet or around a wire conducting electricity. It is sometimes called the etheric aura or the health aura; the Sanskrit term is *prānamāyakosha*, or the vehicle of *prāna*.

Prāna was introduced in lesson 2, p. 17. It is the vital energy which sustains the link between the life of the body and the life of the vehicles of higher consciousness. It also links the individual with the life of the cosmos. It is often translated as the breath of life. Just as we take in oxygen through the lungs to maintain the life of the body, so we take in *prāna* through the skin from the surrounding "psychic atmosphere".

It will therefore be seen why the skin plays an important role in the health of the body. If you sit quietly and feel your consciousness in your skin, you will begin to feel that extension beyond the surface of the skin. Then as you breathe in, think of the idea that you are absorbing *prāna*, vitality, through the whole surface of the arms, the legs, the body, the head. This should produce a sensation that can best be described as an expansion of consciousness.

The sense of touch is the most widely extended sense and embraces all the other four senses, for they have all been evolved from the skin. Sight, smell, taste and hearing are just specializations of the sense of touch. For this reason touch is the most difficult to restrain and the skin should be treated with care. Learn to refine it by feeling, with the fingers, surfaces that are pleasant: velvet, silk, grass, polished wood, artistic shapes.

In lessons 4 and 5 instructions were given for cutting off the senses; this must not become a regular habit, or you will become a day-dreamer, unobservant, "head in the clouds". In this lesson we have indicated how yoga should help you to become more alert, more sensitive.

Sense restraint means control of the senses, not to let them control you. You may suppress them for meditation, but you must also be able to use them when required—to be bright, alert, responsive and observant. At the same time you must keep control so that you do not live just for pleasurable sensation and excitement.

To sum up, learn to use the senses wisely and positively, and when desired to be able to cut them off by an effort of will, as, for example, when meditating, studying or doing any job that requires your full attention.

Concentration (*dhāranā*)

In the last lesson exercises were given for daily practice. For this lesson continue those exercises at the time you have allocated for regular daily yoga practice.

In this practice of concentration, try to avoid the chain association mentioned in the last lesson. An apple was suggested as an object for concentration. The apple may remind you of your apple tree, of the need to prune the tree correctly, last winter you did it in the cold weather, it was snowing, how the children enjoyed the snow. Mary caught a cold, she had to stay away from school, what a nice teacher she has—oh dear! what a long way we have got from our apple! If this happens, try to trace the chain of thought backwards. This exercise will help you to know why your thoughts drifted. So begin again and do not let them drift.

In this lesson suggestions are made for exercises that can be done at any time during the day. They are such that you may make them a regular habit of life, for they will improve your efficiency and your memory. You will be able to add others, particularly some to fit in with your daily life, your business and your leisure time.

The training of the mind in concentration will proceed more quickly if you apply it to your daily life. Pay one-pointed attention to each job you do: writing a letter, baking a cake, reading a report, repairing a machine, making something. If your mind wanders you will probably find that it is because you are thinking about another job that has to be done. You are harassed because you have so much to do that you wonder how it can all be done in time.

Concentrate on one job, and do that well. Later you will be able to supervise more than one job, but you will concentrate all the time, even if only for a brief moment on each job. This is how a mother has to look after her house and her family. She has many jobs, but to each she gives full attention for the immediate moment.

Try the following during the day:

Concentration on a journey. As you walk, note the sequence of the scenery as you go by. The houses, the shops, a special tree and so on. Do this, say, for just one length of a road. Then try to reproduce in memory the order of what you saw.

If it is your regular walk, you can do the same again on the next day, and the next. The practice will not only help in concentration, it will improve your memory.

Selective thinking. During the day, before you begin a new job, think clearly about it. Suppose you are working in the garden. Look at the work you are going to do, digging, or weeding, or pruning. Concentrate on the work ahead, plan the best way to do it, be clear in your mind as to just what you want to do and how you can do it most efficiently. Then proceed—keeping your mind on the job. An efficient workman is one who can keep his mind on what he is doing.

Meditation (*dhyāna*)

As already stated, the term meditation includes all acts of serious and sustained reflection, or mental contemplation. In books on yoga the term is used in the broad sense as including concentration, meditation and contemplation. The Sanskrit word for this is *sanyama*. Ernest Wood (in his book *Yoga*) translates this as poise. The word meditation is used also in a narrow sense to mean continued attention taken beyond the plane of sensuous perception. Here the Sanskrit word is *dhyāna*, the stage between concentration and contemplation.

In this narrow sense meditation is the consideration of a subject in its many aspects and relationships. In concentration we fixed our mind on the subject. In meditation we think around the subject; this is the stage of comprehension, the act of understanding. The subject unfolds before the mind's eye to produce in one's consciousness a deeper meaning because one's attention is taken beyond the level of the five physical senses.

Meditation is a mental process which may be described as "having a discussion with oneself". The subject is considered from all angles until gradually all opinions merge into one comprehensive experience of understanding. The yogi in deep meditation becomes one with the object of his thinking, but he retains his mental consciousness. He thus arrives at an appreciation of reality or truth of that on which he meditates.

In the exercises on meditation, begin with concentration, and then gradually advance to meditation. Concentration contracts the mind and focuses it on the subject. Meditation expands the mind around the subject, enlarging the field of consciousness. Thus concentration is limited to what is placed before the mind's eye; meditation is creative and opens the mind to a deeper understanding of the subject. In order to appreciate this difference it is proposed to begin with concrete objects such as were used in lesson 5 (p. 43).

Meditation on a concrete object. Any one of the objects given in lesson 5 may be taken, but an apple is used here. Begin exactly as described for concentration. When you can hold the apple in thought so that the mind does not wander, then you are ready to meditate on the subject. Think about the relation to other fruit; its distinctive taste, its place in the life-cycle from tree to flower, to fruit and seed, and hence to a new tree; its food value and vitamin content; its place in the scheme of life and the relation between animal and fruit, between the animal and vegetable kingdoms.

As you think around the subject you must not wander away from it. It is as if you allowed the mind to move around the thought of an apple, but always kept the thoughts tied by a mental thread to the apple. This process has been described as an oscillation in thought from the apple to its properties, then back to the apple and out to its uses, and back again to the apple, then out to some other property. After each excursion outwards the mind is brought back again and again to the apple, until every aspect has become part of your consciousness. You will then have identified yourself with the abstract idea or archetype of which the apple is but an outward manifestation.

Five to ten minutes is quite long enough for the exercise, which should be brought to a close in the usual way suggested in the last lesson.

The above type of exercise can be adapted to any concrete object. It has been given as an introduction to meditation in order to show the difference between concentration and meditation. In the next lesson we shall go on to exercises using abstract subjects, leading to self-realization, that is, raising the level of consciousness to that of one's spiritual Self.

Daily Practice

For this lesson your 10–15 minutes of yoga practice should include the following:

53

Body discipline. The relaxation posture.

Breathing. (*a*) The basic breath.

(*b*) Regular rhythmic breathing at, say, 7 seconds in and 7 seconds out.

(*c*) The bellows breath if desired.

Concentration. Continue with the exercises given in lesson 5.

Meditation. Begin meditation exercises as suggested in this lesson.

During the day, practise the following:

Sense restraint. Keep your senses alert as suggested in this lesson.

Concentration. Practise the exercises given in this lesson: on a journey and selective thinking with imagination.

LESSON 7

In the next three lessons we are going to focus our attention on the three internal steps of raja yoga, concentration, meditation and contemplation. It is therefore desirable, before proceeding farther, to recapitulate the five external steps. These were a preparation for the ultimate goal of Self-realization.

Behaviour. Remind yourself of the moral and ethical requirements as given in the five *self-restraints* and the five *self-disciplines* (lessons 1–5).

Body discipline. Have you adopted the personal hygiene and dietary recommendations given in lessons 1, 2 and 4? Have you found your most comfortable posture for meditation (lessons 3 and 4)?

Breathing. Have you improved your intake of the life forces by steady, deep and relaxed breathing (lessons 1–4)? Are you able to find time each morning for the exercises recommended?

Sense restraint. Remind yourself of the suggestions made in lessons 4 and 5 for the control of the senses (sight, smell, taste, hearing and touch) so that they cease to disturb the mind when it is engaged in meditation. Also read again the section in lesson 6 on the wise use of the senses to increase one's powers of response, a valuable asset in preparing for concentration.

Concentration

Lesson 5 (p. 44) included a concentration exercise on a part of the body (an internal object), the example taken being the little finger. This was a preparation for concentration on an occult centre which is used in most forms of yoga.

According to the ancient occult tradition of India, the physical body has associated with it a subtle or ethereal counterpart which is a duplicate of the dense form and extends slightly beyond the surface of the body. It has been called the etheric double and is the vehicle of *prāna*, the vital energy of the cosmos (see p. 17 and p. 48).

The function of this etheric double is to absorb *prāna*, or vitality, and to distribute it to the whole physical body. This is achieved by a number of psychic centres, called in Sanskrit chakras (wheels), which are situated on the surface of the etheric vehicle, about one-quarter of an inch from the skin of the dense physical body. These centres receive *prāna*, which is then distributed over a network of communication to the whole of the physical body with its etheric double, thereby creating fields of vital energy. The whole system serves to link the dense physical body with man's higher principles: his emotional and mental vehicles of consciousness, his spiritual Self and his will, the highest principle of human consciousness (in Sanskrit, *ātma*).

For further details we recommend *The Chakras* by C. W. Leadbeater and *The Etheric Double* by A. E. Powell. For an advanced study see *Serpent Power* by Arthur Avalon. A brief summary is given in the author's *A Simplified Course of Hatha Yoga*, pp. 38–41.

Concentration on an occult centre. There are two occult centres or chakras most often used by raja yogis. One is at the *brow* between the eyebrows (the *ajnā* chakra), which corresponds with our higher Self or that principle of consciousness which may be called "the illumined mind". In theosophical literature this is referred to as *buddhi-manas*: *buddhi* is the harmonizing principle, *manas* in this context is the higher mind. *Buddhi* is sometimes called the intuition, but wisdom is a better translation. *Manas* literally means the mind, but it is always associated either with *buddhi* (the life of the Spirit) or with desire (Sanskrit, *kāma*). Thus *buddhi-manas* is the higher mind illumined by the Self.

The other most used centre is in front of the *heart* and represents the highest principle which controls desire and action.

It is a common practice to begin a meditation by focusing the consciousness either at the *brow centre* or at the *heart centre*; each individual will find which suits him the better. With this object in mind you should now practice concentration on these two centres, one at a time.

Sit in your chosen position, eyes closed, breathing steadily. Feel your consciousness focused between the eyebrows. Think of the brow chakra as a disc, say, of 2–3 inches diameter; the centre of the disc is pulsing with life. Think of vitality, life force (*prāna*) flowing into the centre and filling the mind with a "clarity of thought". The mind is steady, calm, wise, filled with pure thoughts, kind thoughts, a wisdom which transcends ordinary thinking.

The above has taken concentration into meditation. It can lead to an awakening of the intuition, to inspiration.

Proceed slowly, 1 minute only as a beginning, never more than for 5 minutes at a time, and great care must be taken not to be so intense as to produce a headache or feeling of eye-strain or tension anywhere. If you feel a

57

slight warmth in the centre, this is natural, but stop before it becomes too stimulating.

If the exercise makes you feel excited, then you are allowing too much play to your emotions. Keep the exercise at the mental level.

Close the exercise by a few deep breaths, open your eyes with a feeling of being alert and ready to face the world of activity into which you have to go.

A similar exercise may be carried out on the heart chakra, but in this case, after thinking of vitality (*prāna*) flowing into the centre, you will feel (rather than think of) the heart as full of devotion, of love. Here you will not be awakening intuition, but filling your whole being with pure love, pure devotion.

This exercise should be closed by letting your love flow out from the heart centre over the world, to those in need of that spiritual help, whether the need be because of illness, of worry, of distress of any kind, or whether it is that encouragement is needed to carry out an important job as for a school teacher, a doctor, a nurse or a national leader.

Here again care must be taken to proceed slowly and to stop at once if there is any feeling of excitement or if the heart begins to feel as if it is beginning to beat hard or fast. Allowing love to flow outwards is a good relaxation which should avoid the possibility of strain.

Concentration on a quotation or mantra. In lesson 5 the concentration exercises were on concrete objects, both external and internal, and on an idea, as, for example, a virtue. In this lesson we have applied the internal object, such as a part of the human body, to the occult centres of the etheric body or double. An application of the exercise on an idea is to use a quotation, a verse, an invocation or a *mantra*. The quotation may be from the sacred writings of the religions of the world, or from inspirational literature.

The use of such quotations is a regular custom in most meditational practices, but you should begin by using them for the concentration stage, for which purpose a short phrase must be chosen with a clear concise meaning.

It is useful to memorize the quotation in the evening ready for use next morning. The following are just a few examples:

"No man is an island, entire of itself" (*John Donne*, 1571–1631).

"Within you is the light of the world" (*Light on the Path*).

"Kill out all sense of separateness" (ibid).

"I could wish I had often been silent" (*The Imitation of Christ*).

"Blessed are the pure in heart" (*New Testament*).

Sit as usual for your daily practice. Take a few deep breaths. Withdraw the consciousness from the senses. Fix the attention at the mental level and repeat the selected quotation silently to yourself, e.g. "No man is an island".

Concentrate your thought on this idea. You are not on your own. You are part of the human brotherhood. Not alone. Not an island. Not an island. Not isolated.

"No man is an island." Repeat this phrase until it becomes a part of your inner consciousness, part of your mental atmosphere. Gradually it will become the whole of your thought, it will fill your whole consciousness. You will be conscious of nothing else but of the phrase "No man is an island".

Then let the mind relax, open your eyes and let the thoughts of the outside world flow in again.

If you have been successful you will then feel that you now really appreciate the difference between concentration and the mental state of just letting any thought flow into the mind.

The examples given above were ordinary quotations. This exercise can also be used for a *mantra*, that is, a form of words rhythmically arranged so that when sounded they generate vibrations to produce specific effects in higher planes of consciousness. In this case the words are recited aloud and repeated over and over again.

Examples of mantras are:

Sanskrit invocations such as the Gayatri used by Hindus:

> "Om, tat savitur varenyam
> bhargo devasya dhīmahi
> dhiyo yo nah pracodayāt."

(We meditate upon the adorable light of the Creator of the Universe. May he guide our understanding aright.)

The Buddhist invocation in Pali, beginning:

> "Namo Tassa Bhagavato Arahato Sammāsambuddhassa."

(Praise be to the Lord, the Holy One, Perfect in Wisdom.)

The Tibetan *mantra*:

> "Om mani padme hum."

(O, the jewel in the lotus.)

60

The Hebrew invocation to the one Lord:
"Shemāa Yisrael Adonai Elohenu Adonai Eihād."

(Hear, O Israel, the Lord is our God, the Lord is one.)

Latin prayers used by Roman Catholics such as:

"Kyrie eleison, Kyrie eleison, Kyrie eleison,
Christe eleison, Christe eleison, Christe eleison,
Kyrie eleison, Kyrie eleison, Kyrie eleison."

(Lord have mercy upon us, Christ have mercy upon us, Lord have mercy upon us.)

The English translations are given for interest, but they do not have the mantric value of the originals.

Some English invocations and phrases have acquired mantric value by traditional use:

"Holy, holy, holy, Lord God Almighty."

"Glory to God in the Highest, and on earth peace, goodwill toward men."

"Closer is He than breathing, and nearer than hands and feet" (Tennyson).

"There is an inmost centre in us all,
Where truth abides in fullness" (R. Browning).

Mantras are particularly used for mantra yoga (see p. 2), but they can be used as exercises in concentration. What has to be avoided is the constant repetition which can lead to self-hypnosis. In raja yoga it is most important to maintain a positive attitude of mind. Stop whenever you feel yourself drifting into a somnolent state.

Meditation (*dhyāna*)

The meditation stage was introduced in the last lesson with an example using a concrete object—an apple. This example was taken in order to show the difference between concentration and meditation, using the same external object as was used for concentration in lesson 5. Meditation, as generally practised, does not normally use concrete objects; in future you will choose subjects of a more abstract nature.

The Sanskrit word *dhyāna* is derived from the root-verb *dhyai*, to meditate, but its deep significance is that "the mind and heart are bathed in pure knowledge and enlightenment, free from the attractions of the lower world". It is the gateway to eternal contemplation, *samādhi*.

In lesson 5 we took an abstract idea for concentration and specifically concentrated on the virtue of sympathy. This will now be taken to the stage of meditation.

Meditation on a virtue. Begin as you did when concentrating on sympathy, but, having induced an intense feeling of sympathy in yourself, proceed to think around the subject.

Think of people with whom you are in sympathy, because you think along the same lines, belong to the same organization, have common interests.

Then think of those who have quite different views from your own. Can you be in sympathy with them? Although they may differ from you, can you understand their point of view? Recognize that it is possible to be in sympathy with such people.

Sympathy can also be applied to those who suffer, whether such suffering be physical pain or mental anguish. Then realize that in giving them your sympathy you must do it without becoming emotionally involved. Try to understand the meaning of detached sympathy.

Thinking around the subject in this way, you will

gradually bring your thoughts to a focus on the abstract idea of sympathy. Think of sympathy without any specific example, just the abstract idea of sympathy. This is called meditation without seed. The earlier stages were with seed, or with seeds.

You must not try to meditate without seed too early or you will become negative. Always begin with a seed as given in the above example. Later you may be able to meditate without seed, from the beginning. At the present stage proceed as suggested here and allow only a brief instant at the final "without seed" thought. In fact, when you begin the stage of meditation you should stop before you reach the abstract stage. Only add that as you become more proficient.

It is wise to finish a meditation on a virtue by thinking of the qualities of that virtue as spreading out over the world. Thus think of other people around you becoming sympathetic to one another and let this idea spread to embrace your district, your country, the world. And close with a determination to be, yourself, an example of that virtue.

Daily Practice

You should now be laying the foundations for a regular and ordered daily practice.

For this lesson allow yourself 10–15 minutes each day as follows:

(1) *Revise the first five stages of yoga:* behaviour (restraint and discipline), body discipline, breathing and sense restraint. This may be done in the following order:

Body discipline: Relaxation posture.
Breathing: (*a*) Basic breath (this naturally follows the relaxation posture).

63

(*b*) Regular rhythmic breathing at, say, 7 seconds in, 7 seconds out, for six inhalations.

(*c*) You may or may not decide to do the bellows breath; if you do, limit it to six inhalations.

The above should not take more than 4 minutes, at most 5.

Behaviour: Remind yourself of the five *self-restraints* and the five *self-disciplines.* Take one only of these, each day, and it may be a good idea to keep to the one chosen for a week. Then take another for the second week, and so on to cover the ten behaviours every ten weeks. The amount of time you allow for this will depend upon how much time you can spare for your yoga practice. Let us assume 2–3 minutes.

Sense restraint: At this stage you may give a few minutes each day to the restraint of one of the senses, taking them in the order given in lessons 4 and 5. Later you will not need to include this as a separate exercise as it will be done automatically when you begin your meditation.

The above revision of the first five stages of raja yoga can be done in 10 minutes. If you cannot spare more than 5 minutes in order to allow at least 10 minutes for concentration and meditation, then you should do a behaviour *or* a sense restraint each day, and some days you may omit them altogether.

(2) *Concentration* or *Meditation.* Each day do one of the exercises given in this lesson. It would be well to practise concentration for two days and then meditation for the third day. If you allow 5–10 minutes for this

exercise, you should be able to manage your daily raja yoga practice in 15–20 minutes.

It will be necessary to allow at least four weeks for each lesson. This will enable you to have a fair amount of practice in concentration and meditation, even if you only do 5–10 minutes a day on those stages.

LESSON 8

Vehicles of Consciousness

The object of raja yoga is to gain control of one's lower vehicles of consciousness by the highest principle of man, his will. The lower vehicles include the physical body (the body of action), with its vital or etheric double and the mental–emotional or thinking–feeling part of our consciousness. Thus control of the lower vehicles means control of action, feeling and thinking. Feelings or emotions include our desire nature.

The higher consciousness of man is taken to be that part of our nature which operates with abstract ideas, broad views and a clear understanding. As with the lower duality of emotional-thinking, there is a higher duality which is the illumined mind. Here the intellect is replaced by the mind and the feelings or emotions by a principle which has been called the intuition, but is probably better described as inspiration, illumination, understanding.

Above this illumined mind is the will, not the capricious will of a fractious child or of a despot, but the driving force of a well-balanced spirit which achieves its objective by calm perseverance.

As the science of yoga has its origin in the ancient Sanskrit literature, it is of interest to have the Sanskrit terms for the above vehicles or principles of consciousness as the English translations do not always give the full meaning.

Kāma is the desire principle. *Manas* is the thinking principle. So *kāma-manas* with the physical body constitutes man's lower self.

66

Buddhi is the principle in man which gives him spiritual consciousness or enlightenment. *Manas* is dual and can therefore be associated with *kāma*, the feelings, or with *buddhi*, the spiritual aspect. Thus *buddhi-manas* is the Higher Self, or Spirit of man which exists after the death of his lower vehicles.

Ātma is the highest principle of man, the pure Self. It is this which we have called the will in the above introduction to the subject of man's constitution. "Divine will" might give a clearer picture of this highest principle.

This principle, *ātma*, is both universal and individual. Thus man, through his highest principle of *ātma*, is rooted in the Universal Self or Spirit of the universe and yet he also has an individual existence in his own Higher Self. It is the principle of *ātma* which gives *buddhi-manas* an identity as a spiritual consciousness. In that consciousness *ātma* manifests as understanding, judgment, discrimination. We therefore often find the Higher Self referred to as *ātma-buddhi-manas*.

One who has transcended the limitations of the individual Self is a *Mahātma*, beyond *ātma*. His consciousness has merged with the Universal Self.

The above explanation of man's constitution, of his lower self and his Higher Self, has been given because we are now approaching the climax of raja yoga training, the attainment of union with the Real, the Eternal: the opening of the doors of the lower vehicles of consciousness to the power of the Universal Self.

Concentration

Concentration on the Self (Ātma). Seat yourself as usual. Take a few deep breaths. Withdraw consciousness from the senses.

67

Say to yourself—My Real Self is beyond time. I live in the Eternal.

As you repeat these two phrases, feel your consciousness focused at a point within. According to your own inclination this point may be in the region of the heart or in the head. Do not try to think round the subject of the Self, but just feel that point of consciousness which is the master of our whole being.

Now say—I am the Self,
        That Self am I.

And so feel your whole consciousness focused at a point, a point that has neither place nor time.

Do not do this for more than 3 or 4 minutes. Later we shall take this idea into the meditation stage, but at this point of training you are just learning to keep the attention focused on that one idea—the Self, the spark of the divine. If you incline towards Christian practice you can think of "the Christ within" or "the kingdom of Heaven within your heart". In more general terms think of the Self as the inner ruler immortal.

Conclude this exercise by allowing the point of consciousness within to expand again to embrace the whole body with its complex organization, its feelings, its thoughts.

Meditation

The subjects suggested for meditation are those already used for concentration. Thus in lesson 6 we took a concrete external object, such as an apple, which was used for concentration in lesson 5. In lesson 7 we took an idea, such as a virtue, which we used for concentration in lesson 5. In this lesson we shall take a quotation, as used in lesson 7, and then develop the

68

concentration of this lesson 8, on the Self, to the meditation stage.

Meditation on a quotation. In lesson 7 you will have used several quotations for concentration practice. You should now use the same quotations for meditation. Spend a minute or two fixing the attention on the quotation by repeating it several times to yourself and then proceed to develop thoughts about it. What does it mean? What is its deep significance?

Begin by relating the ideas in the quotation to your own life, but then gradually become impersonal, try to understand its significance without any reference to yourself.

Begin by taking the same example used before:

> "No man is an island, entire of itself:
> every man is a piece of the Continent,
> a part of the main."

This is the full quotation from John Donne, but only the first line was used for the concentration exercise in order to keep the mind within limits. For meditation you might now use the whole quotation as you are going to think around the subject.

Pass quickly through the stage of concentration by repeating the phrases until your whole thought is concentrated on them, that is "anchored to them".

Then think about the subject in more detail. An island is surrounded by water, which isolates its inhabitants from the mainland. If I think of myself, my needs, my future, I am like an island separated from other people, not interested in their welfare.

But, no man is an island, so I cannot remain aloof, I must live in association with other people. Their interests are my interests. Their welfare is my concern.

I am not alone, not isolated from other people. They influence me and I influence them. So we should realize our communal interests.

We are all different, but we share a common humanity, a common brotherhood.

Let the thought rest there. Feel that lively interplay between people, between yourself and your neighbours. Embrace them into your consciousness.

You will be able to think around the quotation from many different angles. Let the mind do this, but do not allow it to wander from the main theme. In other words, you can look at the quotation from different points of view, but you never lose sight of the theme of the quotation, you do not wander off into a chain of thoughts which finish up without any clear connection with the original subject.

A meditation such as this can be brought to a close by allowing thoughts of love and understanding to flow towards your whole neighbourhood with a strong feeling that you are an integral and cooperative part of that neighbourhood.

Meditation on the Self. Here also you are going to take the same subject as that used for concentration, and develop your thinking into a meditation. Begin this exercise after you have spent several days in concentration on the Self (*ātma*), as given earlier in this lesson.

When concentrating you avoided thinking *around* the subject. In meditation you ponder upon all aspects before focusing your consciousness on a realization of the whole meaning of the subject. In this case we are aiming at Self-realization with all the hidden power the thought can evoke.

70

You may use the following thoughts as you begin your meditation on the Self, in fact, this form can be used as an introduction to all kinds of meditation.

After sitting relaxed and after taking a few deep breaths, say:

The body is resting (feel it relaxed, rested).

> I am not the body (feel the consciousness withdrawn from the physical body to the vehicle of feeling).

The emotions are calm (feel your emotions losing any excitement, neither elation nor depression).

> I feel love enfolding all.
> But I am not my emotions. (Feel consciousness withdrawn from the vehicle of the emotions. Feel the mind as controller of the feelings and continue:)

The mind is steady. I understand:

> (Here you do not need to say, or think, what you understand: not "I understand other people", nor "I understand what I have been studying or meditating upon", but just "I understand", in the sense of I grasp mentally, I perceive the significance; or put rather colloquially "I know what I am doing". Another way of describing it is that I have removed all uncertainty and so my mind is steady.)

> But I am not the mind.

The Self is wise. The Self controls my thoughts. I am the Self. (At this stage you may think about the

71

Self. Recapitulate in your mind what has been given at the beginning of this lesson about the Higher Self, *buddhi-manas*, and about the highest human principle, the will, *ātma*, and so lead to the climax as follows:

Within me is a divine spark, an inner light. This is the true Self, Eternal, beyond space and time. I am that Self, that Self am I.

The above may be based on the idea of raising the consciousness to higher and higher levels, or of withdrawing consciousness from the outer periphery to an inner centre. Use whichever method comes easier; you may have to try both in order to decide which to use. Whichever method you use, there will come a time when the lower vehicles of consciousness are transcended, and this includes the mind, which means that you cease to think because you just exist, you are, and that will be the initial stage in contemplation.

To come back to the world from such a meditation, think of the Light of the Highest giving illumination to the mind and say:

May my mind be irradiated with wisdom.
May my heart be filled with love.
May my body be strong.

Then take a few deep breaths and come back into full worldly consciousness with the strong sense of an inner power that will rule your day's activities.

Contemplation (*samādhi*)

Samādhi is derived from *sam*, together, and *ādhā*, to direct, hence it literally means to direct together, or to unite. It has been interpreted as to unite lower consciousness or self with higher consciousness or Self, but it really is a state of being completely self-possessed *at all levels*. The consciousness may be raised to the level of man's highest principle, his will or *ātma*, but he takes his lower principles with him. In this sense he does not reject his lower or external links with the outer world but he transmutes them into a "wholeness", a unity of Spirit.

It is said that, in a state of *samādhi*, consciousness with its faculties is collected into oneness or union with the very essence of being, which is even above man's highest principle, above *ātma*.

H. P. Blavatsky defined *samādhi* as "the state in which the ascetic loses the consciousness of every individuality, including his own". This implies that there is not only union between higher and lower but also between the one and the many.

The term contemplation has been used as this has been used in so many books on yoga, but it must be recognized that it requires the amplification given above. This is the eighth step in raja yoga, the goal of our practice. In meditation we tried to reach the essence of the subject chosen. In contemplation we try to experience impersonal awareness of that essence.

In concentration and meditation the mind was applied to the subject, thinking about it. In contemplation we transcend the mind, we cease to think, we become.

This is not easy. We may just enter the stage by a point of our consciousness, but if we think that we are in a state of *samādhi*, then we are no longer there, our consciousness has dropped back to the thinking level. In contemplation we are beyond thought.

Patanjali put this, "When the mind is so far concerned

73

with the object alone, to a degree of one's seeming non-existence, that is *samādhi*" (I, 41). (Free translation by W. B. Gibson, *The Key to Yoga*.)

As this final stage is approached it will be realized that it is going to be difficult to give detailed instructions, as the use of words will necessarily keep the mind active and hold it chained to the outer world. The student must therefore use the following exercises as best he can, and try to achieve an experience rather than an intellectual attainment. Such experience is described as "when all sorrows cease, all miseries vanish, when the seeds for action will be burned, and the soul will be free for ever" (*Raja-Yoga*, Vivekananda).

In view of what has been said above, the exercises on contemplation in this and the next lesson are presented with as few words as possible. Contemplation has been described in most books on the subject as difficult and hard to achieve. Experience shows that it need not be difficult, but this will depend upon the preparation the aspirant has been prepared to do. Do not expect quick results. Make sure of all the preliminary stages, the five preparations and then concentration and meditation. You may try contemplation before perfecting concentration and meditation, but then go back time and time again to the earlier stages. You will be surprised at the final result.

Contemplation using a quotation. First, take any of the quotations used for concentration (lesson 7) or for meditation (in this lesson) and at the close of the meditation stage just stop thinking and experience the fruit of that thinking. In particular, use the quotation "No man is an island", and at the point of "embracing all your neighbours into your consciousness" (p. 70), stop

74

thinking and just experience that broad expansion of consciousness.

Finish the exercise as suggested for that meditation.

The above will introduce you to the idea of what you hope to achieve. It will then be easier, so far as contemplation is concerned, to take more abstract quotations such as:

"I am verily the Boundless."
"As I desire divinity, I become divine."
"Truth is the light of the world."

The first quotation above may be worked out through meditation on our lower vehicles of consciousness as follows. Think of the physical body with its limitations. Then realize how we expand our grasp of the world around us by travel and by reading about other places, by vicarious experience. In this way we begin to understand how we can transcend the limitations of the physical body by the power of thought.

But thought itself has its limitations. We can only think in terms of past experience or of communicated experience. When we think creatively we are expanding our mental consciousness.

Is there a power within us that can transcend thought —a realm, as it were, where there is no conflict of ideas, where all is harmony? Harmony is all-embracing, boundless.

So I am boundless, beyond space, not here, nor there, but everywhere—and at this point cease to think, experience Infinity.

Hold it for a second, perhaps several seconds. Time does not matter in this experience.

Such an exercise, such an experience, needs to be closed slowly by steady breathing, a calm unexcited recollection that we come back to the world to help the world, that we accept limitation that we may help others who are equally limited, limited in their thinking, in their emotional outlets, in their physical surroundings. Think "may we, creatures of this world, find release as we surrender worldly things to the service of the spiritual nature."

Contemplation on a virtue. Take the same example used in lessons 5 and 7, sympathy. Spend a minute or so in concentration on sympathy (lesson 5, p. 44), then about 5 minutes in meditation on the subject (lesson 7, p. 62).

When you have reached the point of meditating without seed (p. 63), just let your consciousness sink into a state of perfect sympathy, an expansion of consciousness that you cannot describe, but only experience. This is an exalted state of feeling best described as an ecstasy of sympathy for the whole of Nature.

This exercise, as with all contemplation exercises, must be brought to a close without allowing the emotions to become involved. In true contemplation, *samādhi*, you are beyond the emotions, just as you are beyond thought. If you can do this exercise impersonally, then you will avoid the danger of an emotional outburst, for it is the personal that overstimulates the emotional nature.

Daily Practice

For the period of this lesson you should work on the concentration, meditation and contemplation exercises given in the lesson, but always begin with the relaxation and breathing exercises.

The main work should be on meditation. This can be

followed by a brief experience in contemplation of the same subject. At this stage of your training you will begin to understand the difference when the mind moves from meditation to contemplation, but do not try to make the change too definite or step-like. Let one merge into the other.

LESSON 9

Contemplation

From what was said in the last lesson and from your experience with the exercises, you will have realized that the subjects for contemplation should be of an abstract nature. Concentration can use any subject from a concrete object to an abstract principle. So can meditation as a technical exercise, although for its practical application it is better to use ideas rather than concrete objects.

The goal of raja yoga is to find the inner Self. "The yogi does not look heavenwards to find God. He knows that HE is within." (*Light on Yoga*, Iyengar). Thus when the yogi reaches the climax of his meditation, he passes into a state of ecstasy where his physical senses and emotive-thinking faculties are quiescent as in sleep and yet his wisdom-understanding is alert. He has transcended thought as such and become an illumined centre of what can best be called supra-consciousness, a vivid, alert dynamo of "energy-standing-still". This is *samādhi*.

It is therefore recommended that the subjects taken for contemplation should be such as will raise the level of consciousness from the mundane world of experience to an inner centre which transcends experience, which is beyond normal consciousness and which is in contact with the Universal Self or life of the Cosmos.

We may think of the Self within as a point of consciousness, but at the same time it embraces the universe —this is why the word supra-consciousness was introduced. Within that Self there is no sense of I or mine.

78

There is only an experience of indescribable joy, a peace beyond understanding, a power which is mightier than all worldly authority. The knower and the known have become one.

Ordinary meditation can and should be used for control of behaviour, for so-called spiritual development, for mental discipline and to open the doors of the mind. But contemplation requires greater intensity at a higher level and so the subjects suggested are usually associated with the Universal Self, with an experience of Bliss, with qualities that are all-embracing in their action.

Contemplation on the Self. Begin as suggested for meditation on the Self (p. 70), that is, omitting the concentration stage.

When the mind has pondered deeply on the idea of the Self, hold it still. The next stage, contemplation, may be regarded as a form of concentration, but at a higher level and without form. Just feel that centre within.

Become the Universal Self.

It has already been stated that these contemplation exercises would necessarily be presented with as few words as possible. If, however, you read the following *before* you begin the meditation, you may be able more easily to get into the atmosphere of what you are trying to do.

Feel the inmost centre of your being as a point of consciousness which is completely withdrawn from all outside contacts. Feel it as a centre through which power from above can flow. Feel your whole consciousness focused at that point. Feel radiant, pure, subtle.

You are now omnipresent, omniscient, omnipotent, but as such you are selfless because you are "All-Self". You are one with the Self of the Universe.

The following quotations will also help to create a realization of the Self:

"The unreal hath no being; the Real never ceaseth to be."

"A wise man abandoneth all the desires of the heart and is satisfied in the Self by the Self."

"The disciplined self, mastered by the Self, goeth to Peace." (The above are adapted from the *Bhagavad Gita*.)

"And now the self is lost in Self,
        thyself unto Thyself,
        merged in That Self,
        from which thou first didst radiate" (*Voice of the Silence*).

"This Spirit within my heart is smaller than a grain of rice, or a grain of barley, or a grain of mustard seed.

And yet it is greater than the earth, greater than the sky, greater than all these worlds" (*Upanishads*).

"The self, harmonized by yoga, seeth the Self in all beings, all beings in the Self; everywhere he seeth the same" (*Bhagavad Gita*).

Contemplation on the impersonal. As for the previous exercise, begin by meditating on the subject. You should by now not need to think about the concentration stage. In future you will practise concentration only as an occasional exercise in order not to forget how to focus attention on a subject. When you begin any meditation, the mere act of choosing the subject should be enough to focus attention on that subject, so you immediately proceed to think round it as an act of meditation.

The impersonal being negative, the mind begins by considering the positive, the personal, that is, pertaining to the person. Me and my possessions. My desires, my thoughts. My prejudices. Me and mine.

But the impersonal means having no personality, no reference to a person, no personal existence or identity, no distinctive personal character.

The impersonal is that shadowy background, behind manifestation, not definitely associated with any particular object or entity.

Follow such thoughts by feeling the very essence of impersonality. Freedom from both possessions and identity.

As for the previous exercise, if you read the following before you begin the meditation, you may be able to enter into the contemplation stage as a natural climax to the meditation.

Feel free as air. You are a spirit. Your own past personal experiences do not influence your present thinking, because you are free from your past. Nor do your future plans influence you; you are free from your future.

You are neither attracted nor repelled by what you see or hear. You are quite impersonal.

The following quotations may also help:

"I seek nothing for the separated self.
I am content to be in the light or in the dark,
to be active or passive,
to work or wait,
to speak or to be silent,
to take praise or reproach,
to feel sorrow or joy."

"In the thoughtless self-less state lies the hidden Spirit of the Universe."

"I am in the world, but not of it."

"Kill out all sense of separateness" (*Light on the Path*).

"Look for the flower to bloom in the silence.

Not till the whole personality of man is dissolved and melted can the bloom open." (Adapted from *Light on the Path*.)

Contemplation on unity. Begin this as a meditation.

Work out your own ideas on unity using the following by way of introduction. Unity or oneness implies that parts of a whole are interconnected and interdependent so that each part shares the life, spirit or existence of the whole, whether that whole be a machine or a group of people.

Unity implies harmony between the parts. Each part has its own function and may be different from every other part. Thus unity does not insist upon uniformity. Particularly apply these ideas to human relations: to the family, the business or factory community, the town, the nation, the world.

Let your thinking reach a climax in feeling unity, not just as an emotional sensation but as an experience beyond emotion or thought. Just be that unity.

You might bring your thinking stage to this climax by saying to yourself, "I am of the nature of fundamental existence, knowledge and bliss, free and self-sufficient, one with all other selves."

Then for one brief instant, heaven opens and the individual becomes one with all other selves, one with the whole world, one with the Supreme Over-self (*parātma*).

Such a meditation, such an experience in contemplation, can be closed by allowing the mind to take up the thought again as an invocation for the whole of humanity to be illumined by that spirit of unity.

"Behold, how joyful a thing it is for all men to dwell together in Unity." Feel that idea radiating outwards to embrace the whole world.

Finally, say to yourself, I now know that unity, I go out into the world to meet my fellow men in that spirit.

An alternative approach

The idea of unity can be taken in an entirely different way. Instead of thinking of the unity as between people, think of the unity within. Harmony between our feelings and actions. Control of the emotions by the mind. An overall harmony of all our vehicles of consciousness from the highest spiritual level.

These suggestions are made to enable you to work out different lines for yourself. Meditation with contemplation cannot be imposed, it must be self-developed until it becomes a background influence throughout the whole day.

Meditation on Helping Others

The following is given as an example of the practical value of meditation.

Throughout the ages individuals and groups of people have used the power of thought for helping others: for healing the sick, for promoting "good causes", for influencing the world for peace and goodwill.

It is a good idea to include such ideas in daily meditation. It helps to keep the practice out-turned, for the service of others and not just for one's own personal spiritual development.

Certain rules must be understood before undertaking this kind of meditation.

With regard to healing, it is better to send thoughts of vital energy to the sick person rather than to think of the specific disease. This means that you do not think of the person with all his aches and pains, but you visualize him as strong and healthy.

In sending help of any sort to a distressed person you must be quite impersonal in your thinking. Do not decide what is good for him, and then try to force the thought on him whether he wants it or not. There must be no sense of compulsion. The thought should be that the person to be helped may be inspired to do what is right for him.

In helping world leaders we must not be partisan. Just think of them as being wise and illumined, and not as taking any specific line of action.

The following is a typical group meditation for the helping of others. The leader of the group reads the phrases slowly and leaves quiet intervals for the members of the group to develop the ideas in their minds.

Begin by sitting in a circle and let each member feel that he is in harmony with all the other members.

Then continue:

"We offer this group to be a channel for the forces of peace and goodwill.

Let us feel ourselves to be in the presence of the Lords of Light and Life and Love.

May their blessing flow into us that we may be the embodiment of peace and goodwill.

May their blessing flow through us to all in authority:

to rulers and heads of government,
to religious leaders,
to all who teach in schools and universities,
to doctors and nurses,
to mothers and fathers.

May their love flow out to all."

Close as follows:

"May our minds be irradiated with wisdom.
May our hearts be filled with love.
May our bodies be strong."

The above example calls upon higher powers. We should, however, have confidence in our capacity to help. One reason for using an expression such as "May we be a channel" is that it helps us to be impersonal. Training in raja yoga should have made us impersonal, so we can "presume to send our blessing", not in the sense of forcing our ideas on others, but as "giving to each as his need is".

You will be able to adapt the example given above to any other form of help for others.

Any group meditation for helping others can of course be adapted for use by an individual in his personal meditation. You may decide to work out a shorter form as a general practice for the concluding stage of your daily individual meditation.

The Raja Yogi

You have now worked through the eight steps of raja yoga from the preliminary moral and ethical improvement of behaviour to the climax in contemplation. What have you achieved and what is the real purpose of this effort?

We have spoken of contemplation, *samādhi*, as the ultimate goal, the final step, the aim and object of all yoga. It is better to realize that all steps are means to an end, not the end in itself. An exercise is always a means; the end is a state of being.

85

What, then, is the state of being a raja yogi? He is one who has control over his thoughts, feelings and actions. He recognizes that man is Spirit, and that the mind and body are his servants. He behaves in harmony with his fellow men, recognizing that all are members of one Human Brotherhood. He is therefore an influence for calm judgment and an inspiration for peace and understanding in any community in which he moves.

He is consciously or subconsciously in tune with the infinite source of Being, and therefore he is able to call upon that source for inspiration and guidance. But such inspiration results in action that is selfless. There is no sense of superiority, no sense of spiritual aloofness; the yogi looks calmly at life in all its aspects.

With this achievement you can be a dynamo of spiritual power.

Daily Practice

For the period of this lesson, work on the contemplation exercises given in the lesson, always doing the relaxation and breathing exercises before, or as an introduction to, the meditation.

Three subjects have been given: the Self, the impersonal and unity. You might work out meditations for yourself on such subjects as: Reality, Love, Harmony, Truth, Sincerity. In each case let there be that brief glimpse of Reality, beyond thought, that brief experience of *samādhi*.

You may also try out the meditation on helping others as an individual meditation.

LESSON 10

Revision and Advice for the Future

This is the last lesson, which means you have completed the training of this simplified Course. It should have taken 10–12 months. How proficient you are in raja yoga will depend on how much time you have been able to give to the practice. The general recommendation is a minimum of one quarter of an hour each day, preferably half an hour.

You should by now have realized the benefit of yoga discipline in the whole of daily life and therefore will wish to continue for the rest of your life. This lesson is devoted to suggestions for revision and for the establishment of a regular daily programme to suit your inclination and circumstances.

Glance through the nine lessons in order to get them into proper perspective and to assess how much you have achieved. You should also decide how much of the whole Course you wish to adopt.

Then decide whether you are ready to proceed with your own planned programme, or whether to go through all the nine lessons once more. Having completed the Course you may feel you went through it too quickly. Also you may feel that, having the full background of the whole Course, you can make a better use of each lesson by starting at the beginning again.

It was pointed out in the Introduction that formal raja yoga comprises eight steps (*āshtānga*), which one is expected to take in the order given. In this Course we have preferred to recommend the aspirant to take several steps concurrently.

Behaviour. This included five *self-restraints* and five *self-disciplines.* The object of these recommendations for moral and ethical control is to ensure that the would-be yogi has control over his conduct before acquiring greater power such as advanced yoga practice will inevitably give him. We have taken five lessons to cover this subject, as steady progress is more easily made if one does not try to embrace too wide a field all at once.

You should realize that the ten injunctions for good behaviour are not all that is expected of the aspirant. They should be regarded as examples of the more obvious aspects of what is required for good behaviour, and they do provide a sound foundation.

For each injunction a key word has been chosen to describe it, such as non-violence for the first self-restraint. In the text alternative translations for the original Sanskrit (in this case, *ahimsā*) have been given, e.g. non-injury, non-killing, not to cause pain physical or mental, or expressed positively as: kindness, helpfulness.

Make your own list of the ten injunctions and choose your own key words to remind yourself of them. In doing this, bear in mind that the five restraints are injunctions of what not to do and the five disciplines are injunctions of what you should do. You may prefer to express all ten as positive affirmations, in fact this is preferred (see p. 6). The reason for giving the restraints in negative form, in the first place, is because this follows the ancient yoga tradition.

Body discipline. Our life here on earth is so much constricted by the limitations of the physical body that we should do what we can to ensure that it may be as healthy and fit as possible, hence the attention to hygiene and diet.

Attention should also be given to adequate physical exercise. In hatha yoga special stretching exercises are included. These are not for muscular development but to give free flow of vitality to the whole body. These exercises are called postures (*āsanas*, see p. 21) because in each case the body bends or stretches into a special position for the free flow of nervous energy. They are not exercises in movement.

In raja yoga the only postures specifically included are those used when meditating, that is, they are different ways for sitting cross-legged on the floor or on a cushion. In this Course we have added a posture not used in traditional Indian yoga practice. This is the Egyptian posture, based on the statues, reliefs and wall-engravings of ancient Egypt. Use the cross-legged posture if it is easy for you, otherwise keep to the Egyptian form.

Breathing. In raja yoga control of breath is limited to the establishment of steady, full and relaxed breathing as a regular habit. There is no need to force a slow rate of breathing, so long as it is regular and rhythmic. Just adopt a rate that is easy and comfortable.

During meditation the breathing will be somewhat slower than this, say up to 7 seconds in, 7 seconds out. Do this for six inhalations before meditation, but then let the lungs take up their own timing. Your thoughts by then will be elsewhere, not on your breathing.

We have also given an idea of the association between breathing and *prāna* according to yogic tradition: *prāna*, the non-physical life principle which pervades the whole universe.

Sense restraint. Control of the five senses is a necessary preliminary for mental control. The senses keep us in constant touch with the world, but their impressions

89

can be over-exciting and sometimes misleading. We must be able to look within, undisturbed by the distractions of the outside world. This we do particularly when performing any mental exercise, such as concentration or meditation.

At other times we have to learn the practical value of the senses, they must therefore be kept alert and sensitive.

Sense restraint in its broadest sense means sense control. This is negative when the mind wishes to be free, and positive when in contact with the world around.

The above five steps of raja yoga are regarded as preliminary and preparatory. They are called the external steps or limbs (*bahiranga*). Their practice leads to disciplined control of the external or lower vehicles of consciousness so that the mind may be free to look within undisturbed by the without.

The first five steps are assumed to have been taken to some degree of proficiency by lesson 6, although one may not feel satisfied until one has repeated those six lessons. Thus it should not be necessary to keep on repeating the five external steps as permanent raja yoga practice; they should be kept in one's consciousness as a background to life. To achieve this state you may occasionally refresh your memory by re-reading in the first seven lessons the sections which deal with behaviour, body discipline, breathing and sense restraint

Breathing and sense restraint will not need much special attention as you will be applying these controls whenever you meditate.

The next three stages in raja yoga are internal (*antaranga*). They operate within the mind. All three are sometimes called by the general term, meditation, but it is usual to specify the stages as concentration, meditation and contemplation. As these words do not fully define the stages, we prefer the Sanskrit terms: *dhāranā*, *dhyāna* and *samādhi*.

Concentration (*dhāranā*). This is the act of focusing one's whole attention on a subject, which may be a concrete object or an abstract idea. We all do this at some time during the day when particularly interested in what is being done or when doing something intricate that requires special attention.

In raja yoga practice it is usual to make a definite exercise of concentration rather than just to rely upon one's normal daily activities. It must, however, be recognized that such exercises are only mental gymnastics and exercise the mind just as physical gymnastics exercise the body of an athlete.

When we become experienced in meditation we do not need to continue concentration as a separate exercise; we automatically concentrate attention on what we are doing, as soon as we begin to meditate. One may, of course, like to do an occasional concentration exercise, just for personal satisfaction, but that will depend on personal inclination.

Meditation (*dhyāna*). This stage will in future be the main daily practice. Those who have established this habit find that meditation in the morning is as necessary for the soul as is food for the body.

In the exercises in lessons 6–9 specific subjects were given for each meditation. It is now suggested that you build up a definite form for your daily meditation by combining several different types of subject to be used as items in a sequence. Suggestions are given here, but it will be better if you later choose your own items and make your own programme. Consider the following four suggestions, try them out, work out alternatives and try them, and finally arrive at your own arrangement. That can then be fitted into the overall daily practice suggested later in this lesson.

I

Make an invocation to the Highest, e.g. "I invoke my Higher Self", or "I open myself to the power of the Supreme *Ātma*."

Create an attitude of devotion, e.g. "I give my devotion to the Great Ones" or "I devote my life to their service." Here you will think of your ideal: the Holy Ones, the Christ, the Lord of the World, the Universal Spirit, the principle of Universal Love, or etc. according to personal belief.

Meditate on a subject chosen for the day (e.g. a virtue, a quotation or an idea).

Evoke within yourself the spirit of that subject.

Give out a blessing based on the subject.

Return to outer consciousness with the thought that the ideas meditated on may be active in your own life.

II

Preparation by reciting a verse from a devotional book.

Withdrawal from the outer world to the Self within. This may be achieved by thinking as follows:

> My physical body is relaxed, at ease, quiet. Pause.
> My restless emotions are becoming quiet, gentle, happy. Pause.
> My mind is quiet, still, calm, serene. It reflects the Peace of the Self. Pause.
> I am the Self. That Self am I.

An effort to contact Reality or some other quality

chosen as the subject (e.g. unity, peace, harmony, or etc.). This is the centre-piece of the meditation and may lead to a brief experience of *samādhi*.

Distribution: thinking of the spirit or essence of Reality radiating outwards to give the world a glimpse of the experience which you have had.

Conclusion. Let the idea (e.g. Reality) illumine your mind, harmonize your emotions, strengthen your body.

(Adapted from a pamphlet on *Group Meditation* by the Theosophical Society in England.)

III

Offering oneself in service.

Invocation. Recite a verse appropriate to the selected high ideal.

Aspiration. Think of that high ideal.

Invocation of blessing. Realize that the Self can experience that high ideal.

Distribution. Let the blessing radiate outwards to others.

Final invocation. Recite again the verse at the beginning.

Suitable verses for the above are:

"What man really seeks is not perfection which is in the future, but fulfilment which is ever in the present."

"To know the not-Self in one's nature is the pathway to knowledge of the Self."

"The meaning of the whole universe is contained in the Self. That Self is in the heart of each man, and it is his very nature to seek that meaning by action and by experience."

"Know for yourself the way along which you should go—do not depend upon others."

93

"In the Spiritual Will there is no coercion of an unwilling self, for the Will is one and moves as a whole."

(From *Thoughts for Aspirants* by N. Sri Ram (Theosophical Publishing House, Madras).)

IV

Fix the mind on the heart centre or at the brow (see p. 56 *et seq*.) and withdraw consciousness from the exterior senses to that centre. This brings the whole body under the control of the will. It is a process of "gathering oneself together". All external feelings are swallowed up in that one central point. You have become "pure mind". This may take only 12 seconds, but you may require a minute or so in the early stages.

Salute your highest; by this is meant saluting with gratitude those who have helped you. An Indian yogi will think of the spiritual teachers of the past and of his own teacher (*guru*). Adapt this idea to your own philosophy of life. You may think of God in the broad sense as the creator or as a personal God; or you may think of a completely impersonal Principle, the God of Immutable Law; or you may think of the One embodied in Man himself:

> Closer is he than breathing and
> nearer than hands and feet.

This is to salute your own highest principle, *ātma*, the Self which is one with the Universal Self.

Choose your own method and salute THAT in a spirit of reverence, gratitude and devotion.

Meditate on the main subject chosen for the day: it may be a virtue, a quality for character building, a quotation, an idea with a spiritual content or any subject of an elevating character. Suggestions have been made throughout the lessons, and earlier in this lesson.

The meditation may lead you into a state of contemplation, *samādhi*, when you will be beyond thought, you will have attained what can best be described as enlightenment on the subject of your meditation. Remain there as long or as short a time as comes naturally; time ceases to matter in that state.

Radiate the blessing you have received over the world. During the meditation you have surrounded yourself with an atmosphere of the subject of the meditation, refined and purified, freed from personal attachment. Let that atmosphere spread out over the world.

Conclusion. Let the consciousness return to the lower vehicles, bringing with it the inspiration you have received. Take a few deep breaths and come back to full consciousness, alert, calm, free from the limitations of worldly desires. Say to yourself: I face the day with equanimity.

Contemplation (*samādhi*). This is the final stage. It is not necessary for all meditation to result in *samādhi*. Meditation, without *samādhi*, is valuable for character building, for awakening the intuition, for seeking illumination or guidance, for helping others. Do not feel that you must always attain the stage of contemplation.

Samādhi more often comes when least expected. If you struggle to reach it, then the disturbance of the mind by that struggling will make it elude your grasp. Some subjects lend themselves more readily to this final stage, particularly those associated with the Self or with Universals.

This brings us to the recognition that the last three stages in raja yoga are really one: concentration, meditation and contemplation merge one into the other, imperceptibly. As you advance in the practice you should begin to drop the distinctions. Do not ask yourself, am I concentrating? am I meditating? Just take your mind along its journey from lower worldly things to higher realms,

> from the unreal to the real,
> from darkness to light,
> from death to immortality,
> (from time to the Eternal),

and do not try to analyse how you are taking that journey.

Typical Daily Practice in Raja Yoga

The following is a suggestion from which you may make your own daily routine. For the meditation stage you can substitute any of the examples (I, II, III or IV) given earlier in this lesson, or any modification of them that suits your temperament. The important point to remember is that our vehicles are creatures of habit and it will therefore help, if you find a form for meditation that suits you, to keep to that form.

On waking, stretch and take a few deep breaths, reminding yourself that you have a day in front of you, which will be filled with joyful activity. You should then be able to rise without reluctance.

After attention to hygiene as suggested in lesson 1 (pp. 9–11), retire to the place you have chosen for your morning yoga exercises. This must be comfortably warm. Then proceed as follows, seated in the posture

96

you have chosen, except for the relaxation exercise and basic breath:

(1) *Behaviour*. Remind yourself of one of the ten behaviours. It is suggested that you take one self-restraint for one week, then one self-discipline for the second week, then the next self-restraint for the third week, and so on to cover the ten behaviours in ten weeks. Repeat this every ten weeks. This recall of the code of behaviour need be only 1 or 2 minutes.

(2) *Relaxation posture* (lesson 1, p. 12) in the prone position. This may take up to 3 or 4 minutes.

(3) *Basic breath* (lesson 1, p. 12) also in the prone position: six breaths, say 1 minute.

Then take your chosen sitting position, making sure to hold the chest, shoulders and head straight and proceed to:

(4) *Regular deep breathing* (lesson 3, p. 23) at four to five full respirations a minute, that is to say 7 seconds inhaling, 7 seconds exhaling. Do this for six full respirations, say 1½ minutes.

The *bellows breath* (lesson 4, p. 29) may be done here if you have time, but this is not essential.

The above, (1)–(4), will take 8–10 minutes. Now proceed at once to meditation which will include sense restraint automatically as soon as you begin.

(5) *Meditation* (concentration, meditation and contemplation). Here you will begin with the programmed sequences suggested, I, II, III and IV, and with alternatives which you may work out for yourself. Eventually you will settle on your final choice. Aim to allow 20 minutes for this meditation stage, making a total of 30 minutes for the *morning yoga practice*.

You may like to include item (1), Behaviour, in the meditation. In that case do it at the beginning: just before the invocation in I or III, before the preparation in II, just before the main subject in IV or make it the main subject.

Remember that raja yoga is not just a once-a-day practice, it is a whole-day way of living. Remind yourself at intervals during the day of the various elevating ideas given throughout this Course.

It is a good idea, at the end of the day, to look back over the day's activities to see where one could have behaved more in line with the high ideals of raja yoga. Such looking back must not be self-deprecatory of the past, but an inspiration for the future.

The Path

In most schools of training for spiritual development one finds reference to a Path, or a Way. In India it has been customary for the aspirant to find a teacher, a *guru*, who will guide his steps along the path towards spiritual enlightenment. The disciple or pupil is called a *chela*. This has resulted in the expression "the path of discipleship" or "chelaship".

One of the oldest metaphors for the growth of the soul is to speak of it as "progress along a path".

In Christianity we find such expressions as:

"Strait is the gate, and narrow is the way, which leadeth unto life, and few there be that find it" (*St Matthew*, vii).

"I am the way, the truth and the life: no man cometh unto the Father but by me" (*St John*, xiv).

"Thou shalt show me the path of life" (*Psalms*, xvi).

"Run the straight race through God's good grace, Christ is the path" (Hymn by J. S. B. Monsell).

98

The Buddhists speak of the noble eightfold Path and "the end of the Path as the threshold of Nirvana".

In the religious philosophy of China, Taoism, the word Tao is variously translated as the Way, the Path, Reason, walking with measured steps in the way of intelligence. "If I have knowledge and resolute faith I shall walk in the Great Tao" (*Tao Teh King*).

The following quotations from theosophical literature give clear meaning to "the Path":

"*The Path*. The Spiritual Way taught in all the great religions, through which man may more swiftly unfold the spiritual powers regarded as latent within him. This is accomplished by the paradoxical process of retreating within and advancing boldly without, by which is meant that as he moves into the depths of his own consciousness he discovers powers and strengths which are then projected into his environment as constructive agencies of the good, the true and the beautiful. The Path is variously termed the Pathway to Perfection, the Path of Perfectibility, the Way of Holiness, the way to Salvation, Liberation, etc. It is considered that all humanity must eventually tread the Path" (*Key Words of the Wisdom Tradition*, L. J. Bendit).

"*The Path*. The pathway is within yourself. There is no other pathway for you individually than the pathway leading ever inwards towards your own inner god. The pathway of another is the same pathway for that other; but it is not your pathway, because your pathway is your Self, as it is for that other one his Self; and yet, wonder of wonders, mystery of mysteries, the Self is the same in all. All tread the same pathway, but each man must tread it himself, and no one can tread it for another; and this pathway leads to unutterable splendour, to unutterable expansion of consciousness, to unthinkable bliss, to perfect peace" (*Occult Glossary*, G. de Purucker).

Such is the goal of true raja yoga. The Teacher to guide our steps is our own Higher Self, the God within.

"Thou art THYSELF the object of thy search" (*The Voice of the Silence*, H. P. Blavatsky).

INDEX

INDEX

104

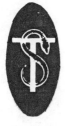